DENTAL SCIENCE, MATERIALS AND TECHNOLOGY

A WINDOW ON SURGERY AND ORTHODONTICS

DENTAL SCIENCE, MATERIALS AND TECHNOLOGY

Additional books in this series can be found on Nova's website under the Series tab.

Additional e-books in this series can be found on Nova's website under the e-book tab.

DENTAL SCIENCE, MATERIALS AND TECHNOLOGY

A WINDOW ON SURGERY AND ORTHODONTICS

GIUSEPPE ALESSANDRO SCARDINA, PH.D.
EDITOR

New York

For permission to use material from this book please contact us:
Telephone 631-231-7269; Fax 631-231-8175
Web Site: http://www. novapublishers.com

Additional color graphics may be available in the e-book version of this book.

Library of Congress Cataloging-in-Publication Data

ISBN: 978-1-62808-948-6

Library of Congress Control Number: 2013947636

Published by Nova Science Publishers, Inc. † New York

Contents

Preface

This book offers comprehensive coverage of new techniques, important developments, and innovative ideas in all fields of clinical dentistry. Some topics discussed in this compilation include the biomechanical considerations of the extraction site in orthodontics; prognosis of operculectomy procedures in vertically impacted mandibular third molars; a 3D analysis of the loop position in anterior retraction arch wire and its effect on produced forces; comparative evaluation of subepithelial connective tissue grafts and acellular dermal matrix grafts in the treatment of gingival recession; understanding and evaluating the role of local anesthesia in dentistry; a review and case report of supernumerary teeth; the biological effects of static magnetic fields of commercial samarium-cobalt orthodontic magnets on cultured escherichia coli and staphylococci aurous; subpedicle connective tissue grafts; surgical removal of genial tubercules; and development of root analogue implants.

Chapter I - In orthodontics, if we would like to achieve the long-term stable dental occlusion within the range of normality and to satisfy precisely our treatment objectives, we have to have long-term stable static and dynamic balanced occlusion within the stomatognathic system. Systematic understanding of orthodontic mechanics and biomechanics is the key stone in this respect. Orthodontics is a very unique specialty dealing with multifactorial phenomena, dental malocclusion, to approach it we have to go methodically to other related fields. The steering signals for successful orthodontics are to be accounted first-of-all with the developing waves of stresses and strains in the periodontium in response to the orthodontic force. Full understanding of the sequence of events in response to the force of occlusion is the key to explore this crucial subject. The objective of this study was to apply basic biomechanical considerations in understanding the influence of extraction of teeth; mesial versus distal to the permanent first molars hoping to open a panel of free discussion in respect of the authors' clinical experience.

Chapter II - *Background:* Impaction of third molars has been assumed to be a sequel to evolutionary changes in humans over the years. However, depending on the circumstances, these third molars may erupt in proper alignment and remain functional, otherwise they remain impacted at different levels and angulations in the jaws, especially so in mandible because of its density and topography. Partially impacted teeth often present with pericoronitis leading to dilemma in diagnosis and treatment options, as to whether to extract or to carry out operculectomy (and retain the tooth). However, operculectomy would be preferred over extraction owing to its conservative approach. But there has been no data available regarding successful outcome of operculectomy in retaining partially impacted teeth. So, the present pilot study aims to evaluate the outcome of operculectomy in class II position I vertically impacted mandibular molars (most commonly prevalent cases posing diagnostic and treatment dilemma). *Materials and method:* 12 patients with 5 of class I (control) and 7 of class II (experimental) impactions were included. They were treated with operculectomy and the degree of occlusal tissue clearance pre-operatively, one week and one month post-operatively was compared using divider and vernier caliper. *Results and observations*: Although statistically significant amount of tissue regrowth was observed in experimental group, there was definite relief of symptoms in the post-operative period. *Conclusion:* Operculectomy procedure can be a predictable procedure in class II position I vertically impacted mandibular third molars in achieving sufficient occlusal clearance. Thus, the clinicians can conserve these impacted molars by operculectomy.

Chapter III - Reducing an increased overjet is an acceptable reason to start an orthodontic treatment to improve esthetics and function of the teeth. Different techniques and disciplines have explained anterior retraction according to their goals and appliance designs. One to ten percent of Caucasian orthodontic patients have one or two missing lateral incisors. [1] Achieving esthetic, functional and long-term stable results in orthodontic treatment of these patients require controlled crown and root movements of remaining teeth.

Chapter IV - *Aims:* To clinically evaluate and compare efficacy of acellular dermal matrix allograft and sub epithelial connective tissue graft in the treatment of gingival recession. *Methods:* A randomized clinical trial was conducted where twenty eight patients presenting gingival recession $\leq$ 4 mm were treated for recession coverage and received either acellular dermal matrix (ADM) or sub epithelial connective tissue (CTG). Prior to and at the end of 3, 6 and 9 months the parameters assessed were: plaque index(PI), gingival index(GI), probing depth(PD), recession depth(RD), relative attachment level(RAL) and width of keratinized tissue(KT). The percentage of root coverage was also calculated and data were statistically analyzed by student's paired t test. *Results:* Both groups yielded improvements in PI, GI, RD decrease, gain in RAL and gain in width of keratinized tissue. The root coverage was 56. 32 % for ADM group and 72. 78 % for CTG group respectively. CTG group produced a greater increase in all the evaluated parameters compared to ADM group. *Conclusion:* The present data appeared to indicate that subepithelial connective tissue graft group showed better clinical improvements than acellular dermal matrix graft group in all the parameters assessed.

Chapter V - Local anesthesia forms the major part of pain-control techniques in dentistry. The prevention and elimination of pain during dental treatment has benefited patients, their doctors, and dental hygienists, enabling the dental profession to make tremendous therapeutic advances that would otherwise have been impossible. Introduced in the late 1940s, the amide local anesthetics represent the most used drugs in dentistry. Local anesthetics also represent the safest and most effective drugs in all of medicine for the prevention and management of pain. They are also accompanied by various adverse effects which should be well known and be able to controlled by the clinician. The article reviews the types of agents uses as local anesthetics and their effects on the human body.

Chapter VI - Supernumerary tooth (ST) is a developmental anomaly and has been argued to arise from multiple aetiologies. These teeth may remain embedded in the alveolar bone or can erupt into the oral cavity. When it remains embedded, it may cause disturbance to the developing teeth. The erupted ST might cause aesthetic and/or functional problems especially if it is situated in the maxillary anterior region. This case involves an 8-year-old male with inverted tuberculate rudimentary right ST located in midpalate region and a left ST erupted palatal to left maxillary central incisor.

Chapter VII - *Objective:* The current study aimed to investigate the biological effects of the static magnetic fields of commercially available orthodontic samarium-cobalt (SmCo5) magnets on cultured two types of bacteria (E-coli and Staphylococci aurous) *Materials and methods*: The study was conducted on: 1. Orthodontic magnets arranged in couples; some of them were fixed in attraction mode and others were fixed in repelling mode with a distance of a 1. 5mm between pole of each two magnets. 2. Three sterilized glass laboratory dishes were plated with Escherichia coli (E. coli) bacteria and another three dishes were plated with Staphylococci aurous. One dish in each group was used as a control group, while the other two dish were used as a test group. On the lid of each test dish, a couple of orthodontic magnets were fixed, one in the attraction mode and the second in repelling mode. 3. The biological effects of the static magnetic field under the two conditions, repelling and attraction modes were evaluated after 48 hours. 4. The above motioned steps were repeated for 9 times. *Results:* 1. The static magnetic field affected significantly the cell populations in different ways according to the type of cultured cells. 2. The biological effects of the static magnetic field in attraction mode were significantly greater than that recorded in magnets' repelling mode. *Conclusion:* 1. Exposure to the static magnetic field of orthodontic magnets for only 48 hours could dramatically affect the growth of Staphylococcus aurous and E-Coli bacteria. 2. The adverse effects of the static magnetic field were significantly higher in attraction mode than that with magnets in repelling mode.

Chapter VIII - *Background:* Root coverage is the goal of periodontal plastic surgery when treating gingival recession. This article describes the use of Subpedicle Connective Tissue Graft (SPCTG) as a bilaminar reconstructive procedure for root coverage. The success of this graft has been attributed to the double blood supply at the recipient site from the underlying bone base and the overlying recipient flap. *Method:* The operation SPCTG was performed on 15 sites with an isolated gingival recession accompanied by an absence of attached gingiva. The connective tissue graft was obtained from palate at premolar-molar area. All patients were evaluated at 7,15,30,60 and 90 days post-operatively. *Results:* From the analysis of results, statistically highly significant root coverage was obtained at 90 days with the mean gain of 84. 66%. The mean area of gingival recession was reduced from 8. 2 $mm^2 \pm 2.\ 99\ mm^2$ to 1. 83 $mm^2 \pm 3.\ 11\ mm^2$. ($p<0.\ 001$). Statistically significant increase in the width of attached gingiva was also obtained with the mean gain of 4. 6 mm. The mean width of attached gingiva was increased from o mm ±o mm to 4. 6 mm ±1. 25 mm ($p<0.\ 01$). *Conclusions:* Based on the results, the SPCTG technique showed high predictability in the treatment of single recession.

Chapter IX - Genial tubercles are tiny bone projections located bilaterally around the lingual foramen, on the lingual face of the mandible. *Purpose:* This study intends to present diagnosis methods and surgical techniques to treat this relatively uncommon problem. *Patient:* A totally edentulous, 69 year old, female patient came to the authors' clinic complaining of an increase in volume in the floor of the mouth, in the region of the lower central incisors, that was causing instability in the lower total prosthesis. Immediate placement with conventional cylindrical implants into extraction sockets has many disadvantages owing to the incongruence of the implant to the extraction socket resulting in a void adjacent to the head of the implant. The purpose of this article is to review the developments that have taken place in root-analogue implants over years including, how various implant materials, implant fabrication and implant placement techniques for root-analogue implants have evolved with time. *Results:* The surgical planning was the removal of genial tubercle, one week after the surgery no one complication was observed. *Conclusion:* Surgical removal of genial tubercles are a rare situation however in this case this surgery was necessary and no complications was observed after the surgery.

Chapter X - Transverse hinge axis is defined as, an imaginary line around which the mandible may rotate within the sagittal plane. Mandibular movements around this horizontal axis is an opening and closing motion and are referred to as a hinge movement. The hinge movement is probably the only example of mandibular activity in which pure rotational movement occurs. A lot of discussion has taken place in past over mandibular hinge axis. The dental profession recognizes the importance of hinge axis. A thorough understanding of various concepts involved in hinge axis is of prime importance. The purpose of this article is to give a complete overview about everything that one needs to know about hinge axis including different types and methods of locating hinge axis and its clinical application in prosthodontic treatment. A PubMed search of English literature was conducted up to January 2010 using the terms related to hing axis. Additionally, the bibliographies of 5 previous reviews, their cross references as well as articles published in dental journals were manually searched.

Chapter XI - Esthetically correct treatment of a localized alveolar ridge defect is a frequent prosthetic challenge. Such defects can be overcome not only by a variety of prosthetic means, but also by several periodontal surgical techniques, notably soft tissue augmentations. This article describes a technique for the improvement of esthetics with conditioning of the tissue beneath the pontics. The technique describes a procedure where a free connective tissue graft is used for augmenting the localized ridge defect followed by a metal ceramic restoration enhancing the esthetics, function and comfort.

Chapter XII - Immediate placement with conventional cylindrical implants into extraction sockets has many disadvantages owing to the incongruence of the implant to the extraction socket resulting in a void adjacent to the head of the implant. The purpose of this article is to review the developments that have taken place in root-analogue implants over years including, how various implant materials, implant fabrication and implant placement techniques for root-analogue implants have evolved with time.

Chapter XIII - *Objective:* The current study aimed to investigate the biological effects of the static magnetic fields of commercially available orthodontic samarium-cobalt (SmCo5) magnets on cultured human lymphocyte cells. *Materials and methods:* To study the effect of the static magnetic field, in attraction and repelling modes, on human lymphocyte cells, two couples of orthodontic magnets were used. One couple was fixed with the magnets in attraction mode and the second one; the two magnets were fixed in repelling mode. On the other hand, three autoclaved glass laboratory tubes were prepared and filled with cultured human lymphocyte cells. One tube was used as a control sample and the other two were used as test samples. Each couple of the prepared orthodontic magnets was threaded into silk thread, immersed and positioned exactly in the center of the cultured lymphocytes. Modified comet assay was used to evaluate the biological effects of exposing the human lymphocyte cells for 48 hours to the static magnetic field of orthodontic magnets under repelling and attraction modes. *Results:* 1. The percentage of DNA fragmented human lymphocyte cells recorded statistically significant level ($P \leq 0.\ 001$) after exposure for 48 hours to the static magnetic field of orthodontic magnets. 2. The adverse biological effects of the static magnetic field in attraction mode were significantly higher than that recorded in magnets' repelling mode. *Conclusion:* 1. Short time exposure (48 hours) of human lymphocyte cells to the static magnetic field of the commercially used orthodontic samarium-cobalt (SmCo5) magnets will end with significant DNA fragmentation of those cells. 2. The static magnetic field of magnets fixed in attraction mode has significantly higher adverse biological effects compared to that fixed in repelling mode. 3. Iron is important dynamic to augment that effect.

Chapter XIV - *Aim.* The treatment of temporomandibular joint (TMJ) ankylosis aims to eliminate the neoformed tissue and to re-establish the mandibular functionality. The purpose of this article is to evaluate the best surgical treatment considering the complications, the functional and aesthetic aspect, through a retrospective study carried out on nine patients treated by resection of ankylosed bone followed by reconstruction with a total joint prosthesis. *Methods.* From June 2003 to June 2009, nine patients presenting with temporomandibular ankylosis underwent a surgical reconstruction of the TMJ by employing a "Quinn prosthesis", at the Department of Maxillary-Facial Surgery of the "Civico" Hospital in Palermo. Among them, 7 were male (25 to 50 years old with a mean age of 42,3) and 2 were female (37 and 54 years old and the mean age was 45,5). *Results.* In the considered sample of patients the mean preoperative maximum interincisal distance was 6,6 mm, this was increased to a mean of 32 mm postoperatively. Only one patient developed an infection postoperatively. *Conclusions.* The authors concluded that reconstruction with a total alloplastic joint prosthesis has proven to lead to successful outcomes in the management of severe anatomic joint disease in adult patients.

Chapter XV - articaine and 2% lidocaine, both containing 1:100,000 epinephrine, and the influence on heart rate during endodontic treatment. *Methodology:* The study examined 244 patients requiring root canal treatment who were randomly assigned either articaine or lidocaine. Anesthetic efficacy was evaluated by the need for additional injections and by self-perceived information on pain reported at several time points on a Visual Analogue Scale (VAS) (total pain perception, pain during injection, and pain during treatment). Heart rate was electronically measured before treatment, during injection, and during treatment. *Results:* Lidocaine was administered to 128 patients and articaine to 116. No statistical difference was found in the requirement for additional injections. The articaine group reported less pain on VAS at all time points ($p<0.005$). A statistically significant difference was observed in heart rate after lidocaine (84. 63 beats/min) compared to articaine (81. 63 beats/min) ($p=0.048$). *Conclusion:* Articaine resulted in less self-reported pain during endodontic treatment.

In: A Window on Surgery and Orthodontics
Editor: Giuseppe Alessandro Scardina
ISBN: 978-1-62808-948-6

Chapter I

Biomechanical Consideration to the Extraction Site in Orthodontics: A Theoretical Approach

Hussam M. Abdel-Kader*
Faculty of Dental Medicine,
AlAzhar University and Misr International University,
Cairo, Egypt

Abstract

In orthodontics, if we would like to achieve the long-term stable dental occlusion within the range of normality and to satisfy precisely our treatment objectives, we have to have long-term stable static and dynamic balanced occlusion within the stomatognathic system. Systematic understanding of orthodontic mechanics and biomechanics is the key stone in this respect. Orthodontics is a very unique specialty dealing with multifactorial phenomena, dental malocclusion, to approach it we have to go methodically to other related fields. The steering signals for successful orthodontics are to be accounted first-of-all with the developing waves of stresses and strains in the periodontium in response to the orthodontic force. Full understanding of the sequence of events in response to the force of occlusion is the key to explore this crucial subject. The objective of this study was to apply basic biomechanical considerations in understanding the influence of extraction of teeth; mesial versus distal to the permanent first molars hoping to open a panel of free discussion in respect of our clinical experience.

Keywords: Orthodontics, Extraction, Biomechanics

* Corresponding author: hmkader@hotmail.com.

"It is good to have static dental occlusion within the range of accepted norm. But it is a challenge to have long-term stable functional dental occlusion. To achieve it; is an excellence in our very unique profession, orthodontics. " Abdel-Kader H. M.

It was stated that "Each tooth lives in its own unique sea of outside forces, moving in response to every shifting, changing influence. So long as we are alive the only stability of tooth position is the dynamic stability of a delicate balance between the many varied forces. "[1] When the force of occlusion acts on the inclined plane of teeth' cusps (canines through molars), it will end for simplicity, into two force's components; horizontal and-vertical components. The upper and lower vertical force components are opposite and more or less equal stabilizing the vertical position of teeth and sufficient enough to resist overeruption of teeth. On the other hand, the horizontal force components are distributed in wave forms all over the surfaces of the inclined planes of the cusps, with the mesial and lingual components are the most dominant. This force distribution affects the upper and lower teeth simultaneously in a similar way, ending with the teeth from the canines through molars tipped forward and inclined lingually in ascending constant harmonized scheme. This pattern allows proper occlusion of the posterior teeth and proper contact area between teeth in the same arch as well as to that in the opposite arch.

To realize the above mentioned statements we have to appreciate them from the mechanical and biomechanical point of view.

It was stated that "Applying a force to anybody has potential effects in directions other than that in which it is applied." [1]. From the mechanical point of view, if the horizontal force components' of the force of occlusion (F); will end with tipping forces whatever in lingual or mesial direction, acts on a lever arm (L) which is the distance from the points of occlusal force application on the inclined plane of the cusp to the center of rotation (resistance) located axially on the root, or at the bifurcation of the roots in multirooted tooth, will produce a moments equal to FL, which is the tendency of the tooth to move around a given point. These movement moments are resisted by equal and parallel forces (R) acting in the opposite directions coming from the supporting tissues of the tooth. These resistant forces R will produce moments equal to RL'; where L' is equal to the distance from the alveolar crest of the tooth investing tissue to the level of its apex. [2] The resistance moment of a tooth is supported by succession of resistance moments of the neighbor teeth, like a ring in chain [3]. The difference between the sum of the external moments resulting from the force of occlusion and all the resistance moments from the supporting tissues must come to zero for the teeth to remain at rest and in tight contact with each other (FL=RL'). The moments of the right and left side of the two dental arches met each other at the central line, are equal and opposite in direction to have harmonious central line of the maxillary and-mandibular dental arches. At any given moment during mastication the two dental arches are in state of dynamic balance. The reverse is true during rest periods, the two dental arches are considered to be in a state of static balance. Accordingly tooth/teeth movements, if any, are the resultant of unbalanced two side of the equation.

From the biomechanical point of view, the periodontium of the teeth experience and transmit the different mechanical stresses generated in response to the force of occlusion. The periodontium absorb, and transmit mechanical stresses generated from either different functional activity of the teeth such as mastication to the basal bone. Mechanical stresses experienced in the periodontium are capable of modulating the soundness and development of this very vital system. Since mechanical stresses transmit through bone, their effects are experienced in a hierarchical manner sequentially as tissue-level bone strain, interstitial fluid flow that in turn induces cell-level strain on bone cells. Periodontal mechanical stresses in response to the force of occlusion are complex because of momentary changes in force direction, muscle function, complex periodontium forms, and the different occlusal surface topography of the teeth and their cusps. Strain patterns vary between different periodontium depending on the number, shape and surface topography of their roots. Adjacent periodontium can experience characteristic tensile or compressive stresses. Mechanical waveforms of the force of occlusion, such as static and dynamic waves at various frequencies are expressed as corresponding stress waveforms and strain in the periodontium. The periodontium absorb large mechanical stresses during mastication either in tension or compression waves. Mechanical stresses during mastication are not transmitted in the periodontium as a continuing gradient, the different periodontium are capable of redefining a propagating mechanical force into predominantly tensile or compressive strain. The periodontal mechanoreceptor is the key in this crucial issue. Normal muscular pressure of the masticatory muscles, normal forces of the inclined planes in mastication and in occlusion, normal interproximal contacts of teeth in the same arch and to that in the opposite arch and harmony in the size of the two dental arches to permit the teeth, in their respective arch, to occupy their position in the line of occlusion are very important dominant factors in this respect [4].

Mastication is carried on by a force-linked closed functional system of muscles, tempromandibular articulation, other bones of the craniofacial complex and teeth. There is a feedback mechanism in mandibular function in which the force exerted by the mandible is fed back again to the jawbone and muscle of mastication, from there back again to the teeth. Since the teeth are a part of the closed force-linked functional system their position are limited to certain area within this system. This area is termed the area of functional tolerance. Teeth within this area will remain stable because they are situated so that they conform to the trajectorial forces generated in function. [4] At any given moment during mastication the two dental arches are in state of dynamic balance. The reverse is true during rest periods, the two dental arches are considered to be in state of static balance. The forces produced by mastication aid in the forward and lateral growth of the dentition and help to maintain the force of the proximal contact of teeth. The orbicularis oris and its associate muscle, in conjunction with the buccinator mechanism prevent the dention from being carried too far forward and laterally. Each tooth in addition to its function in mastication is an essential key in the dynamic balance of the adjacent teeth in the respective arch and to that in the opposite arch, in conclusion the denture position. The dentition reached an apparently fixed form and position, within the craniofacial complex, when all of the forces acting upon it are in state of balance.

The developing waveforms of tensile and compressive stresses in the periodontium, of the different teeth in one dental arch, concomitant to the force of occlusion during mastication, intermingled with each other forming strong chain of tensile and compressive stresses ending within the basal arch of that jaw as called by Salzmann and which Tweed refer to as “the basal bone” [4]. The basal arch which is the stress concentrated area of the jaw structure is located at more or less concentrated portion of the jaw subjacent and superjacent to the alveolar process in the mandible and the maxilla respectively.

Histological examination [5] of the jaw bone reveled that it is formed of three distinctive layer of Haversian system; the first layer is the alveolar bone supporting the teeth, the third layer forming the main bulk of the respective jaw both are formed of many more or less small round Haversian system. While the second layer which is the intermediate layer between the other two layers, is formed of relatively much less Haversian system which are larger in size and oval in shape, as it is compressed between the other two layers. The dimensions of the Haversian system (Osteones) reflect the strength of the bone; it stronger when it is composed of larger and less number of Osteones [6] On the other hand, as a result of these very complexes generated stresses, the bone trabeculae of the respective jaw are arranged and thickened into well defined ridges in order to compensate with the very powerful force of occlusion, which could come to an average of 1500 gm/cm2 root surface area. This special arrangement of bone trabeculae is known as the "Trajectories of force" which indicate the directions of functional stresses within the stomatognathic system [4] .

After the above introduction we have the very important and vital questions in orthodontics; first, what is the effect of extraction of the tooth/teeth on the above mentioned strong chain of mechanics and resultant biomechanics? Second, is there any difference if the extraction is anterior or posterior to the first permanent molars? Third if the nonextraction protocol is the appropriate treatment modality to preserve the soundness of the force of occlusion, periodontium and concomitantly the stomatognathic system in general? It is stated that; the maximum biting force that an individual can generate is dependent on the intrinsic muscular power and pain threshold. On the contrary, a decrease in tactile sensibility as a result of reduced periodontal mechanoreceptors due to extraction of tooth (teeth), may allow an increase in the biting force of the individual [7] To satisfy the six keys of normal dental occlusion as proposed by Andrews [8], in orthodontics, we have to have more respect to the related mechanics and biomechanics. We have to treat our orthodontic patients professionally; putting in consideration that dental malocclusion is actually a multifactorial phenomena.

In extraction orthodontic protocol, the extraction of the four first premolars as the teeth of choice for the orthodontists will end with dramatic reduction in the periodontal mechanoreceptors. In another ward two complete unites are taken out of the periodontium continuous intermingled chain of waveforms of tensile and compressive stresses in their respective arch. In this way the chain will be broken down in very receptive areas in the dental arch, the junction between the anterior teeth segment and the posterior teeth segment, as if we have removed the two key stones from a Gothic arch. At that moment you can imagine the dramatic changes which could be happened in the soundness of the periodontium tensile and compressive intermingled wave-chain of each respective dental arch. The periodontal mechanical stresses in response to the force of occlusion are complex because of the momentary changes in force direction, muscle function, complex periodontium forms in relation to respective roots, and the different occlusal surface topography of the teeth and their cusps, extraction of teeth will be reflected fundamentally on this vital tissue phenomenon. In accordance the static and dynamic balance of the dental arches will be affected.

Other factors have to be in consideration in this respect; first the reduction in the periodontal mechanoreceptors concomitant to the extraction of the four first premolars will radically reduce the perceptible sensibility and increasing the biting force of the concerned patient. This could be reflected adversely on the soundness of the periodontium and subsequently the long-term stability of orthodontic treatment outcome. Second the

Transseptal fibers between the adjacent teeth and the force of interproximal contact. During retraction of the canine through the first premolar extraction space, the transseptal fibers mesial and distal to the orthodontically moved canine will show different degrees of coiling, compression and stretching [9, 10, 3] The rebound inherent tendencies of coiled, compressed and stretched Transseptal fibers will act against maintaining the tight proximal contact between orthodontically approximated teeth, from second premolar to second premolar. [11,12] On the other hand Retain [13, 14] among others [15-19] stated that; transseptal fibers in the supra-alveolar tissues will not show rearrangement and remodeling even after long-retention period, to the extent that surgical transaction of the supra-alveolar tissues, after the active phase of orthodontic treatment, is recommended to reduce strong tendency to relapse.

The second alternative is the extraction of teeth distal to the first permanent molars. Extraction of the molars, especially the third molars is considered successfully in much orthodontic treatment protocol. It was stated that

> "Distalization of the first molars will create enough space along the dental arch to deal with different types of dental malocclusion and malrelation. Under such circumstances, the decision of extraction of teeth will be shifted from the segment mesial to the first molars to the segment distal to the first molars, and extraction of the second or third molars could be selected. Following this method will save the integrity of the dental arch from first molar-to-first molar; from the esthetic, functional occlusion, normal intercuspation, and normal interproximal contacts between teeth. Accordingly, we will achieve long-term stability of orthodontic treatment". [20]

This conclusion is in accordance with other investigators who concluded that; extraction of premolars could end with retroclination of the upper incisors, deepening of the bite, reduce the vertical dimension and over-retraction of the premaxilla. They recommended that to relief crowding required extraction, it was not the premolars, but the second molars that should be removed [21].

The picture is simulating the condition in the nonextraction orthodontic treatment protocol, in which the periodontal mechanoreceptors are preserved; subsequently the perceptible sensibility and the biting forces will be kept at their appropriate level. On the other hand the periodontium strong continuous intermingled chain of mechanical waveforms of tensile and compressive stresses in their respective arch will be kept at their fitting level. Subsequently at any given moment during function or at rest, the two dental arches are in state of dynamic balance or static balance respectively. In this regards we have to be clear that overexpansion of the dental arches to create space in favor of nonextraction orthodontic protocol, will end by distraction of the above mentioned multifaceted dynamic and-static balance of the dental occlusion within the stomatognathic system and subsequently the long-term stability of orthodontic treatment outcome could be very questionable.

In conclusion; extraction of teeth distal to the first permanent molars could be of choice from the biomechanical point if we are looking for:

1. Saving the integrity of the dental arch from first molar-to-first molar; from the esthetic, functional occlusion, normal intercuspation, and normal interproximal contacts between teeth;
2. Achieving long-term stable static and dynamic balanced occlusion within the stomatognathic system.

References

[1] Thurow RC. Atlas of orthodontic principles. CV Mosby USA 1970; 9.

[2] Richter EJ, Orschall B, Jovanovic SA. Dental implant abutment resembling the two-phase tooth mobility. *J. Biomech* 1990; 23: 297-306.

[3] Abdel-Kader HM. Orthodontic canine retraction and concomitant incisor teeth retraction. *Al-Azhar Dent J.* 1992; 7: 97-104.

[4] Grabber TM. *Orthodontics principles and practice*. W. B. Saunders USA 1972; 559.

[5] Abdel-kader HM, Ibrahim SA, Ahmed MH. The basal arch of Salzmann "The stresses concentrated unite of the jaw structure" A histological study. *Al-Azhar J. Dent Science* 1999; 2: 181-5.

[6] Salzmann JA. Practice of orthodontics. *J. B Lippincott USA* 1966; 50.

[7] Richter EJ. Basic biomechanics of dental implants in prosthetic dentistry. *J. Prosthet Dent.* 1989; 61: 602-609.

[8] Andrew LF. The six keys to normal occlusion. *Am. J. Orthod.* 1972; 62: 296-309.

[9] Erikson EH, Kaplan K, Aisenterg MS. Orthodontics and Transseptal fibers. *Am. J. Orthod.* 1945; 31: 1-20.

[10] Keitan K. Tissue rearrangement during retention of orthodontically rotated teeth. *Angle Orthod. J.* 1959; 29: 105-13.

[11] Southard TE, Southerd KA, Tolley EA. Periodontal cause of relapse. *Am. J. Orthod. Dentofacial Orthop* 1992; 101: 221-7.

[12] Abdel-Kader HM, Ibrahim SA. Transseptal fiber system compressive force (TCF) and extraction orthodontics. *Al-Azhar Dent J.* 1993; 8: 679-86.

[13] Reitan K. Tissue rearrangement of orthodontically rotated teeth. *Angle Orthod* 1975; 29: 105-13.

[14] Reitan K. Clinical and histological observation on tooth movement during and after orthodontic treatment. *Am. J. Orthod.* 1967; 53: 721-45.

[15] Erikson BK, Kaplan H, Aisenbas MS. Orthodontics and transseptal fibers. *Am. J. Orthod* and Oral *Surgery* 1945; 31: 1-20.

[16] Thampsen HE, Myers HI, Waterman JM, Flanagan VD. Preliminary microscopic observation concerning the potentiality of supra-alveolar callegenous fibers in orthodontics. *Am. J. Orthod* 1958; 44: 185.

[17] Thampson HE. Orthodontic relapse analyzed in a study of connective tissue fibers. Am *J. Orthod* 1959; 45: 93-109.

[18] Boese LR. Increased stability of orthodontically rotated teeth following gingivectomy in Macaca nemestrina. *Am. J. Orthod.* 1969; 56; 273-90.

[19] Brain WF. The effect of surgical transaction of free gingival fibers on the regression of orthodontically rotated treatment in dogs. *Am. J. Orthod.* 1969; 55: 50-70.

[20] Abdel-Kader HM. Angle's classification of dental malocclusion: Is it capable of new modification and interpretation? *Orthodontic Waves J.* 2010; 69: 82-8.

[21] Witzing JW, Saphl TJ. *The clinical management of basic maxillofacial orthopedic appliances*. PSG Publishing 1987: 156.

In: A Window on Surgery and Orthodontics
Editor: Giuseppe Alessandro Scardina
ISBN: 978-1-62808-948-6

Chapter II

Prognosis of Operculectomy Procedure in Vertically Impacted Mandibular Third Molars - A Clinical Evaluation

Simran Parwani*[*,1], I. K. Kanteshwari[1], Rajkumar Parwani[2] and P. J. Chitnis[3]

[1]Department of Periodontics,
Modern Dental College and Reseach Centre, Indore, India
[2]Department of Oral and Maxillo-facial Pathology,
Modern Dental College and Reseach Centre, Indore, India
[3]Department of Periodontics, YMT College and Hospital,
Yerla Medical Trust, Kharghar, Navi Mumbai, India

Abstract

Background: Impaction of third molars has been assumed to be a sequel to evolutionary changes in humans over the years. However, depending on the circumstances, these third molars may erupt in proper alignment and remain functional, otherwise they remain impacted at different levels and angulations in the jaws, especially so in mandible because of its density and topography. Partially impacted teeth often present with pericoronitis leading to dilemma in diagnosis and treatment options, as to whether to extract or to carry out operculectomy (and retain the tooth). However, operculectomy would be preferred over extraction owing to its conservative approach. But there has been no data available regarding successful outcome of operculectomy in retaining partially impacted teeth. So, the present pilot study aims to evaluate the

[*] Address for correspondence: Dr. Simran Parwani, A-306 Staff Quarters, Modern Dental College campus, Bijasan road, Gandhinagar, Indore-453112 (M.P.), India. Tel. no. +91 9977132697, Fax no. +91 07312882699, E-mail: dr_rnparu@yahoo.co.in.

outcome of operculectomy in class II position I vertically impacted mandibular molars (most commonly prevalent cases posing diagnostic and treatment dilemma).

Materials and method: 12 patients with 5 of class I (control) and 7 of class II (experimental) impactions were included. They were treated with operculectomy and the degree of occlusal tissue clearance pre-operatively, one week and one month post-operatively was compared using divider and vernier caliper.

Results and observations: Although statistically significant amount of tissue regrowth was observed in experimental group, there was definite relief of symptoms in the post-operative period.

Conclusion: Operculectomy procedure can be a predictable procedure in class II position I vertically impacted mandibular third molars in achieving sufficient occlusal clearance. Thus, the clinicians can conserve these impacted molars by operculectomy.

Clinical Significance

Scientific rationale for the study: Scientific literature reported till date describes the treatment of vertically impacted class II position I mandibular molars as extraction. But there is hardly any data as regards the success of operculectomy in retaining these teeth. So, the present pilot study aimed to clinically evaluate the outcome of operculectomy in making these teeth functionally useful.

Principal findings: Significant amount of occlusal tissue clearance was observed after operculectomy in class II position I vertically impacted mandibular third molars. A definite relief from symptoms (of pain and inflammation) was also observed in the post-operative period.

Practical implications: Operculectomy can be a predictable procedure in treatment of class II position I vertically impacted mandibular third molars. Thus, clinicians can conserve these impacted molars by operculectomy.

Keywords: Mandibular third molars, operculectomy, extraction, vertically impacted

Introduction

An impacted tooth is the one, which fails to either erupt partially or totally in its normal place in the mouth due to inadequate space and obstruction by an adjacent tooth or teeth / soft tissue and bone, beyond its chronological age of eruption. [1] Few teeth are more predisposed to impaction than the others due to lack of space in the jaw. Mandibular third molars are usually impacted if the space between the mandibular second molar and anterior border of ramus is insufficient. The soft tissue that covers the occlusal surface of partially erupted mandibular third molar is known as operculum. [2] Operculum is particularly vulnerable to irritation and is often directly traumatized when it is caught between the crown of the tooth that it covers and antagonist tooth during closure of mouth (while eating or swallowing). [3]

The crypt form of the pericoronal tissues favors entrapment of food debris and proliferation of micro-organisms in this area. These factors predispose to acute infections like necrotizing ulcerative gingivitis or clinical condition like pericoronitis. [3]

Pericoronitis is defined as an acute infection with accompanying inflammation of gingiva and contiguous soft tissues about the crown of an incompletely erupted tooth. [3, 4] Most frequently affected teeth are mandibular third molars due to lack of space in the jaw. [5, 6]

The microbial flora that develops in the distally located pseudopocket is the major cause. This flora is predominantly anaerobic i. e., Peptostreptococcus, P. gingivalis, P. intermedius, F. nucleatum. [7-14] Symptoms of pericoronitis include: painful, swollen gingivae in the area of the affected tooth and bad smell or taste in the mouth. In advanced stages, discharge of pus from the gingivae near the tooth and lymphadenopathy may also be present. [15]

Impacted mandibular third molars can be categorized based on two classifications [4, 16, 17]:

1. Winter's classification (1926):
   Vertical, mesio-oblique, horizontal and disto-angular impactions.
2. Pell and Gregory's classification (1933) figure 1 (ref. [18]: Most frequently used classification which is based on 3 criteria –
   A) Availability of space between distal aspect of mandibular second molar and ramus (horizontal plane):
      Class I – Sufficient space to accommodate the mesio-distal diameter of impacted tooth.
      Class II – Space is less than the mesio-distal diameter of impacted tooth.
      Class III – No space is available and hence, entire tooth is buried in the ramus.
   B) Relative depth of the mandibular third molar (vertical plane):
      Position I – The highest point of the impacted tooth is in level with the occlusal plane of the mandibular second molar.
      Position II – The highest point of the impacted tooth is lower than the occlusal plane but above the cervical line of the mandibular second molar.
      Position III – The highest point of the impacted tooth is below the cervical line of the mandibular second molar.
   C) Long axis of the impacted mandibular third molar in relation to the long axis of the mandibular second molar (angulation):
      Vertical, mesio-oblique, horizontal, disto-angular, inversion, linguo-version and bucco-version.
   D) *Management:* The soft tissue impaction can be treated surgically by removing the overlying operculum. This can be done with either a scalpel blade or electrocautery after controlling acute infection. This procedure is referred to as operculectomy. [19, 20]

Indications for operculectomy procedure in soft tissue impacted mandibular third molars [16, 21]:

1. Availability of space for eruption of third molar.
2. Presence and proper alignment of antagonist tooth.
3. Proper alignment of impacted mandibular third molar in the arch.
4. Angulation of impacted mandibular third molar in relation to long axis of second molar – vertical angulation is favourable.
5. The position / depth of the third molar in mandible – position I is ideal.
6. Prosthetic consideration: Requirement of the third molar as an abutment for fixed prosthesis.
7. Socio-economic reasons / patient not willing for extraction.

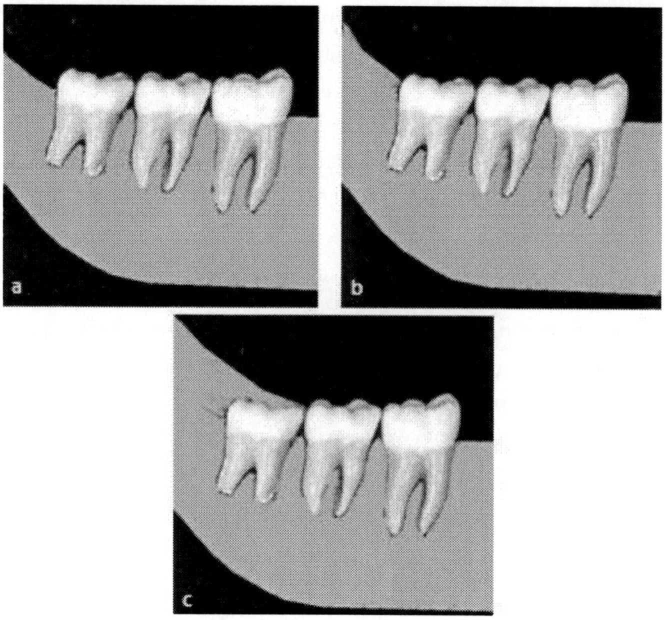

Figure 1. Schematic presentation of different classes of vertically impacted mandibular third molars in position I. Figure 1a: Class I; Figure 1b: Class II; Figure 1c: Class III.

Reason for avoiding mandibular third molar extraction would be that it is associated with morbidity even in routine cases including the lost working time, iatrogenic injury and complications (pain and swelling). [22]

All classes of mandibular third molar impactions other than vertical impactions have to be referred for extraction. Amongst vertical impactions, class III cases have to be referred for extraction at the outset itself whereas class I cases can be successfully treated by operculectomy in order for normal functioning of the tooth. The dilemma lies only with vertically impacted class II cases as regards to the choice of treatment modality. This dilemma led to the curiosity for the present study.

In the present study, a case control trial was conducted, where the patients were selected based on the Pell and Gregory's classification of impacted mandibular third molars. Selection of patients and allocation into test and control groups was done clinically along with the help of intra-oral peri-apical radiographs.

Aims and Objectives

1. Prognosis of operculectomy procedure on class I position I (group I) and class II position I (group II) vertically impacted mandibular third molars was assessed by comparing objective and subjective symptoms (such as bleeding, tissue inflammation / swelling and pain) pre-operatively and post-operatively.
2. To compare the degree of occlusal tissue clearance and tissue regrowth following operculectomy between group I and group II.

Materials and Method

The present clinical trial comprised of 12 patients selected from out-patient dept. of Periodontics, Modern Dental College and Research Centre, Indore; who were included in the study after obtaining their informed consent for operculectomy. The protocol of the study was approved by the ethical committee of the instituition. Patients were divided into two groups with the help of clinical examination and intra-oral peri-apical radiograph, criteria for division being the Pell and Gregory's classification.

Group I (control group) comprised of vertically impacted mandibular third molars in class I and position I.

Group II (study group) comprised of vertically impacted mandibular third molars in class II and position I.

Five patients belonged to group I and 7 patients belonged to group II.

Inclusion Criteria: Systemically healthy subjects in the age range of 17-30 years.

Exclusion Criteria: Class III cases, angulation of impacted mandibular third molar other than vertical, malaligned teeth, presence of trismus, teeth without antagonist.

Clinical Examination: A complete case history of each of the 12 patients was recorded so as to fulfill the inclusion and exclusion criteria. Investigations included intra-oral peri-apical radiograph and haemogram. Grouping of teeth into group I and group II was based on clinical and radiographic analysis.

Clinically the distance from mesial proximal ridge of mandibular third molar to the tip of the operculum was measured with a divider and recorded as "occlusal tissue clearance". This measurement was then placed on a vernier caliper for precise recording. After complete oral prophylaxis, patients were prepared for operculectomy. Pre-operative photographs were also taken to assess the soft tissue coverage over the impacted tooth clinically.

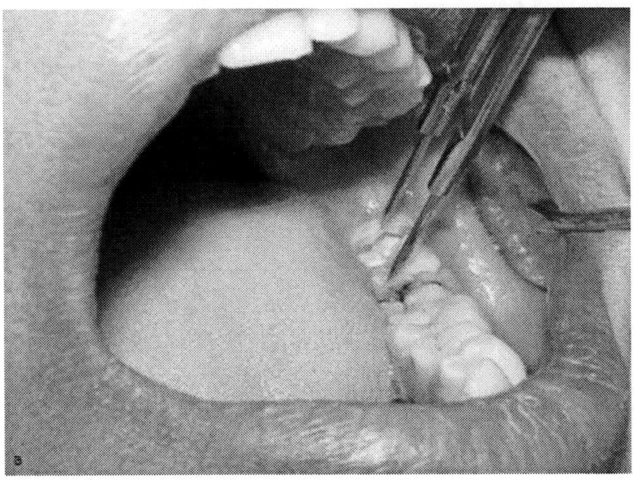

Figure 2a. Assessment of occlusal tissue clearance. Measurement of occlusal tissue clearance with divider.

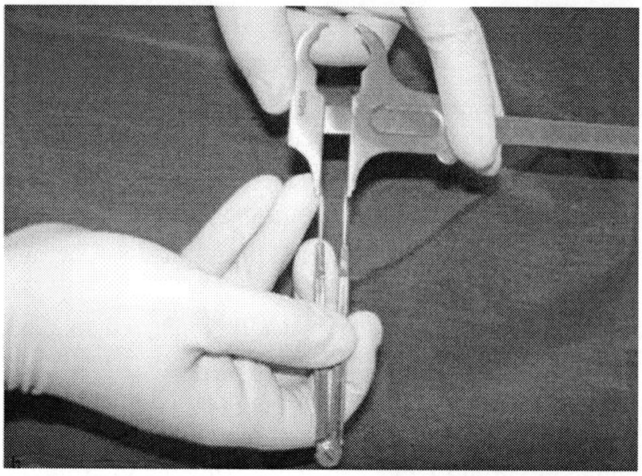

Figure 2b. Assessment of occlusal tissue clearance. Transfer of measurement to vernier caliper.

Assessment of occlusal tissue clearance following operculectomy: (figure 2) Operculectomy procedure was performed with scalpel method to achieve complete tissue clearance on occlusal table of soft tissue impacted mandibular third molar. The occlusal table thus exposed was then subjected to the measurement of mesio-distal dimension using a vernier caliper device. Post-operative photographs were repeated. All patients were prescribed with an antibiotic and analgesic as per the need in individual case. Post-operative instructions were delivered. Patients were recalled after one week and one month. The assessment of occlusal tissue clearance and photographs were repeated.

Case Reports

Figures 3 and 4 depict group I and group II cases respectively with pre-operative clinical view, IOPA, immediate post-operative, one week post-operative and one month post-operative clinical views. These figures show occlusal tissue clearance achieved after operculectomy and the amount of tissue regrowth in the post-operative period.

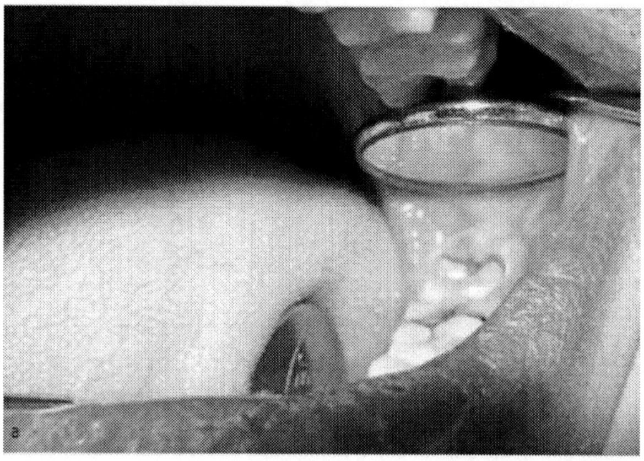

Figure 3a. Case report depicting operculectomy in group I case. Pre-operative view.

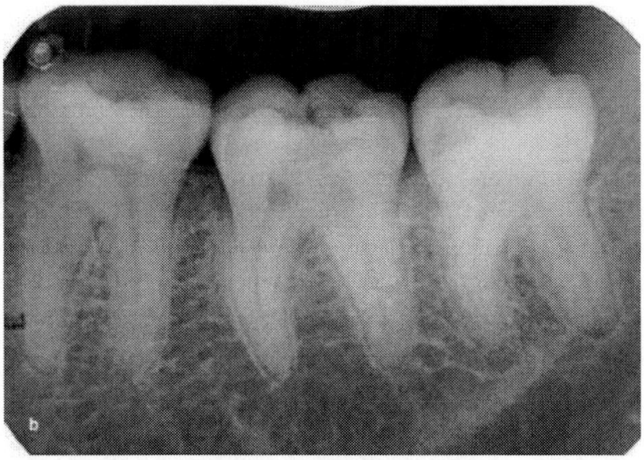

Figure 3s. Case report depicting operculectomy in group I case. IOPA.

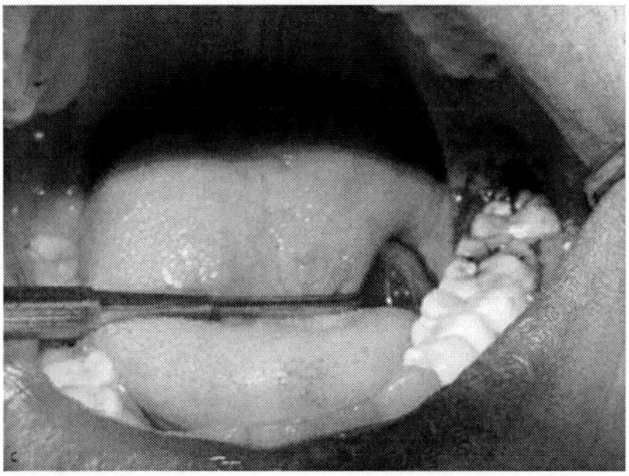

Figure 3c. Case report depicting operculectomy in group I case. : Immediate post-operative view.

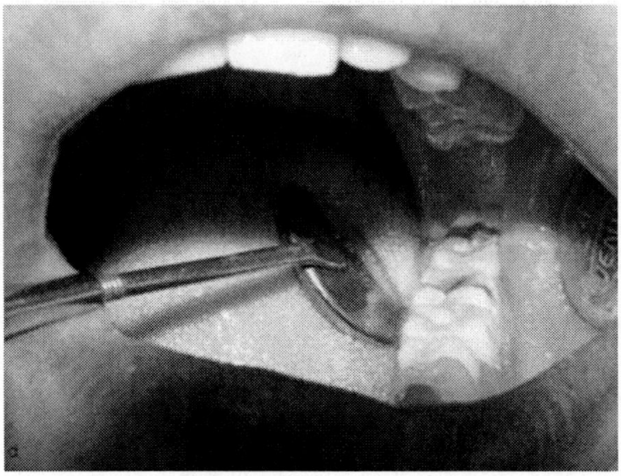

Figure 3d. Case report depicting operculectomy in group I case. 1 week post-operative view.

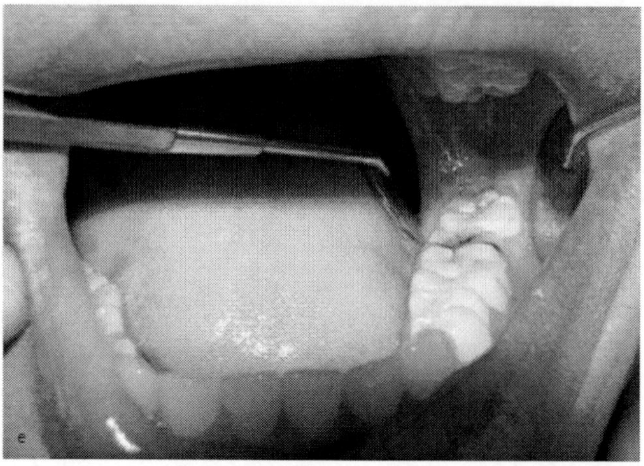

Figure 3e. Case report depicting operculectomy in group I case. 1 month post-operative view.

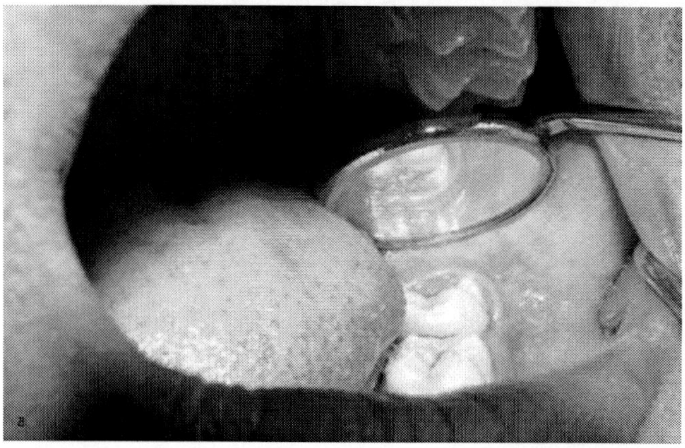

Figure 4a. Case report depicting operculectomy in group II case. Pre-operative view.

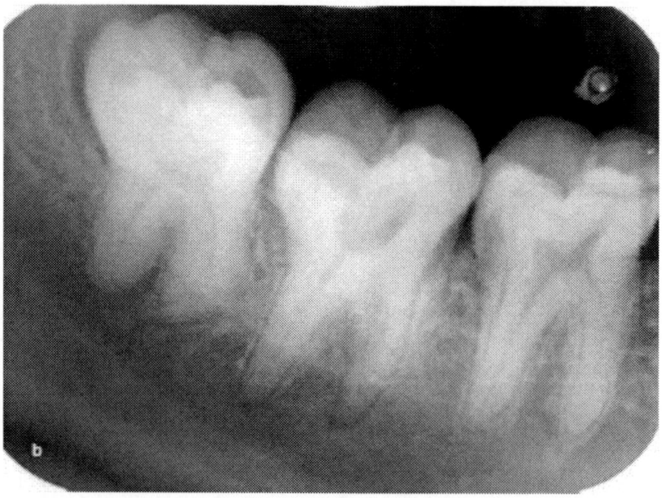

Figure 4b. Case report depicting operculectomy in group II case. IOPA.

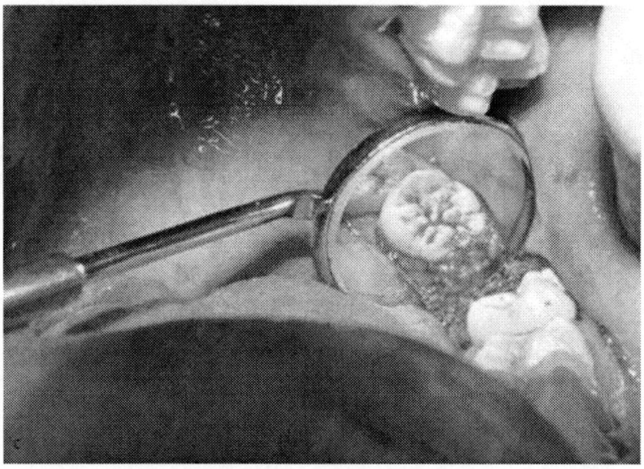

Figure 4c. Case report depicting operculectomy in group II case. Immediate post-operative view.

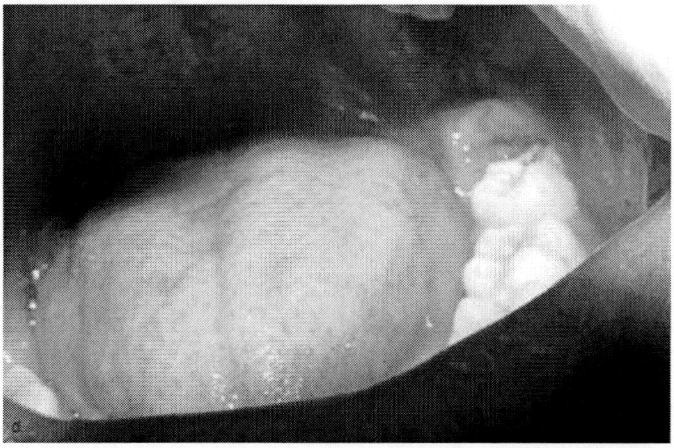

Figure 4d. Case report depicting operculectomy in group II case. 1 week post-operative view.

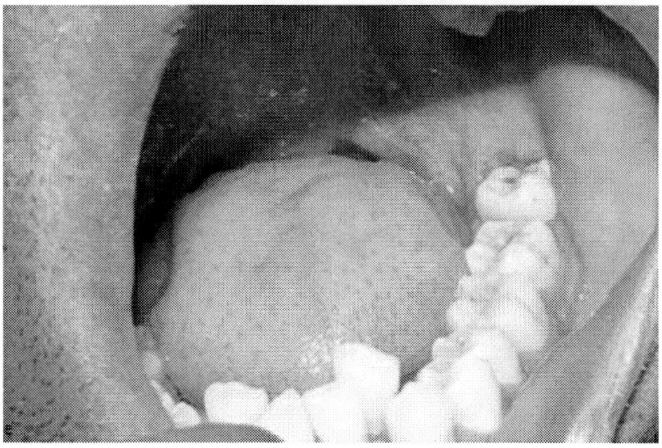

Figure 4e. Case report depicting operculectomy in group II case. 1 month post-operative view.

Results

Table no. 1 shows the comparison of occlusal tissue clearance in group I cases. Pre-operative measurements were compared with immediate, one week and one month post-operative values. Similarly, table no. 2 shows these values in group II cases. Table no. 3 shows the degree of relapse and percentage of operculum tissue regrowth in group I and group II cases at different post-operative periods. Group I cases showed no relapse one week and one month post-operatively as compared to the immediate post-operative values. Paired 't' test was done to evaluate the difference in the post-operative values at different periods in group II cases. Bar graph shows the occlusal tissue clearance in group II cases comparing pre-operative, immediate, one week and one month post-operative values.

Table 1. Comparison of occlusal tissue clearance (in mm) in group I cases

Sr. no.	Pre-operative	Post - operative		
		Immediate	1 week	1 month
1	6. 8	8. 5	8. 5	8. 5
2	6. 6	8. 7	8. 7	8. 7
3	10	11. 5	11. 5	11. 5
4	7. 8	9. 3	9. 3	9. 3
5	6. 9	7. 8	7. 8	7. 8
Mean	7. 62	9. 16	9. 16	9. 16
S. D.	1. 40	1. 41	1. 41	1. 41

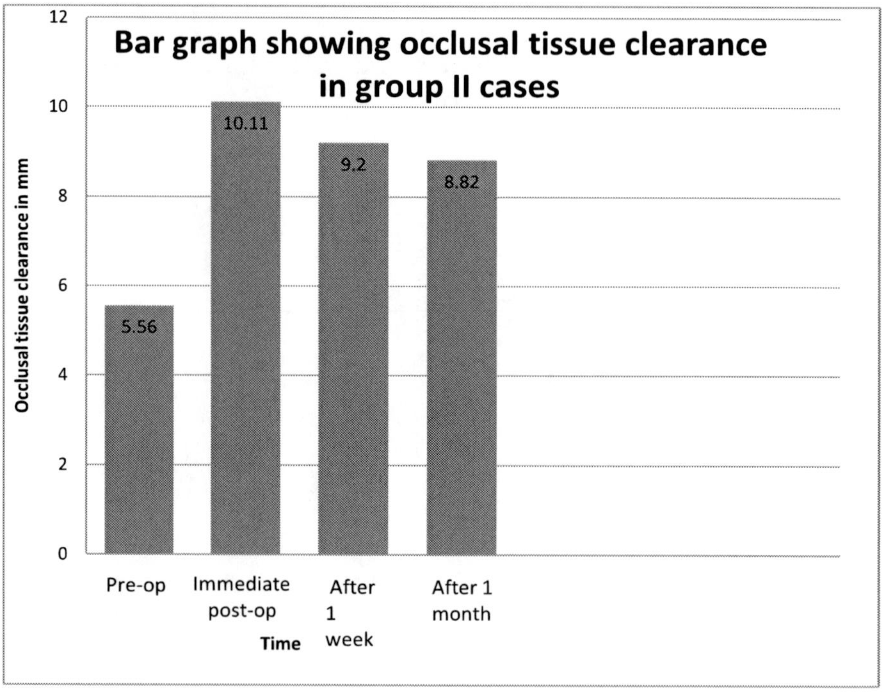

Graph 1.

Discussion

As evident from table no. 1, one week and one month post-operative operculum tissue regrowth was 0%, thus degree of relapse was nil. This implied that the class I position I vertically impacted mandibular third molars can be successfully retained by operculectomy procedure.

From table no. 2 and 3, it is evident that post-operative operculum tissue regrowth was 10% after one week and 13% after one month in group II cases. Maximum amount of tissue regrowth occurred within the first week of postoperative period (10%) and the further regrowth (by 3%) during following one month was clinically not considerable. This regrowth in group II cases at one week and one month follow-up, as compared to immediate post-operative value was statistically significant (p-value 0. 049 and 0. 009 respectively).

Table 2. Comparison of occlusal tissue clearance (in mm) in group II cases

Sr. no.	Pre-operative	Post - operative		
		Immediate	1 week	1 month
1	4. 9	9. 2	9. 2	7. 2
2	8. 2	13. 1	11. 4	12. 1
3	3. 4	9. 3	9. 3	8. 1
4	7. 1	10. 1	9. 0	8. 9
5	2. 6	9. 9	6. 6	6. 7
6	5. 9	11. 7	11. 7	11. 7
7	6. 8	7. 5	7. 2	7. 1
Mean	5. 56	10. 11	9. 2	8. 82
S. D.	2. 03	1. 81	1. 91	2. 22

Table 3. Degree of tissue relapse following operculectomy in group I and group II cases

	Group I		Group II	
	Degree of relapse	Percentage of tissue regrowth	p-value (significance) and degree of relapse	Percentage of tissue regrowth
Immediate post-op. v/s 1 week	No relapse observed	0 %	0. 049 relapse - statistically significant	10 %
Immediate post-op. v/s 1 month	No relapse observed	0 %	0. 009 relapse - statistically significant	13 %
1 week post-op. v/s 1 month	No relapse observed	0 %	0. 161 relapse - Not significant	3 %

($p < 0.05$: statistically significant).

Tissue clearance obtained in group II cases was clinically considerable although total clearance was not obtained in many cases. But, none of the patients experienced discomfort or pain in the post-operative period much against what they did pre-operatively. This implied that the regrown operculum tissue which was left over on the distal surface of vertically impacted class II, position I mandibular third molars was clinically insignificant to be impinged upon / yield to trauma or infection by the antagonist maxillary third molars.

Conclusion

Operculectomy procedure can be a successful treatment plan for class II position I vertically impacted mandibular third molars. It helps to increase the area of the occlusal table. Such teeth can function well, provided that their distal surface is not too close to anterior border of ramus that may jeopardize the width of attached gingiva or they have not been complicated by extraoral swelling and / or trismus. However, results of this study could have been more conclusive if the follow-up was extended to 6 or 12 months and if the sample size were larger.

Acknowledgments

We are extremely grateful to Dr. Ravi Shiratti (MDS in Community Dentistry) for his main contribution in biostatistical work of this study. We also express our heartfelt thanks to the teaching, non-teaching staff and patients of the dept. of Periodontics, Modern Dental College and Research Centre, Indore for their co-operation.

References

[1] Ghosh PK. Impaction. In: Ghosh PK. *Synopsis of Oral and Maxillofacial Surgery*. New Delhi (India): Jaypee Brothers; 2006. p. 14.

[2] Peterson LJ. Principles of Management of Impacted Teeth. In: Peterson LJ, Ellis E, Hupp JR, Tucker MR. *Contemporary Oral and Maxillofacial Surgery*. 4th ed. St. Louis: Mosby (Elsevier); 2003. p. 187.

[3] Grant DA, Stern IB, Listgarten MA. Pericoronitis. In: Grant DA, Stern IB, Listgarten MA. *Periodontics*. 6th ed. St. Louis: The C. V. Mosby Co. ; 1988. p. 421.

[4] Fragiskos FD. Surgical Extraction of Impacted Teeth. In: Fragiskos FD. *Oral Surgery*. New York: Springer; 2007. p. 122-7.

[5] Killoy WJ. Treatment of Periodontal Abscesses. In: Genco RJ, Goldman HM and Cohen DW. *Contemporary Periodontics*. St. Louis: C. V. Mosby Co. ; 1990. p. 479.

[6] Schuster GS. The Microbiology of Oral and Maxillofacial Infections. In: Topazian RG and Goldberg MH. *Oral and Maxillofacial Infections*. 3rd ed. Philadelphia: W. B. Saunders Co. ; 1994. p. 68.

[7] Peterson LJ. Principles of Antibiotic Therapy. In: Topazian RG and Goldberg MH. *Oral and Maxillofacial Infections*. 3rd ed. Philadelphia: W. B. Saunders Co. ; 1994. p. 184.
[8] Blakey GH, White RP, Offenbacher JrS, Phillips C, Delano EO, Maynor G. Clinical/ biological outcomes of treatment for pericoronitis. *J. Oral Maxillofac Surg* 1996; 54: 1150-60.
[9] Leung WK, Theilade E, Comfort MB, Lim PL. Microbiology of the pericoronal pouch in mandibular thied molar pericoronitis. *Oral Microbiol Immunol* 1993; 8: 306-12.
[10] Mombelli A, Buser D, Lang NP, Berthold H. Suspected periodontopathogens in erupting third molar sites of periodontally healthy individuals. *J. Clin. Periodontol* 1990; 17: 48-54.
[11] Peltroche-Llacsahuanga H, Reichhart E, Schmitt W, Lutticken R, Haase G. Investigation of infectious organisms causing pericoronitis of the mandibular third molar. *J. Oral Maxillofac Surg* 2000; 58: 611-6.
[12] Rajasuo A, Jousimies-Somer H, Savolainen S, Leppanen J, Murtomaa H, Meurman JH. Bacteriologic findings in tonsillitis and pericoronitis. *Clin. Infect Dis*. 1996; 23: 51-60.
[13] Sixou JL, Magaud C, Jolivet-Gougeon A, Cormier M, Bonnaure-Mallet M. Microbiology of mandibular third molar pericoronitis: incidence of beta-lactamase-producing bacteria. *Oral Surg. Oral Med. Oral Pathol Oral Radiol Endod* 2003; 95: 655-9.
[14] Wade WG, Gray AR, Absi EG, Barker GR. Predominant cultivable flora in pericoronitis. *Oral Microbiol Immunol* 1991; 6: 310-2.
[15] Pericoronitis [Internet]. Revised 5/2010; Avaivable from: http://www. ada. org/
[16] Srinivasan B. Impacted Teeth. In: Srinivasan B. *Textbook of Oral and Maxillofacial Surgery*. 2nd ed. New Delhi (India): Elsevier publication; 2004. p. 97-9.
[17] Peterson LJ. Principles of Management of Impacted Teeth. In: Peterson LJ, Ellis E, Hupp JR, Tucker MR. *Contemporary Oral and Maxillofacial Surgery*. 4th ed. St. Louis: Mosby (Elsevier); 2003. p. 193-7.
[18] Andreasen JO, Petersen JK, Svendsen H. The Impacted Mandibular Third Molar. In: Andreasen JO, Petersen JK and Laskin DM. *Textbook and Color Atlas of Tooth impactions*. St. Louis, Missouri: Mosby; 1997. p. 264.
[19] Dym H. Management of Impacted Third Molar Teeth. In: Dym H, Ogle OE. *Atlas of Minor Oral Surgery*. Philadelphia: W. B. Saunders Co. ; 2001. p. 83.
[20] Klokkevold PR. Treatment of Acute Gingival Disease. In: Newman MG, Takei HH, Carranza FA. *Carranza's Clinical Periodontology*. 9th ed. Philadelphia: Saunders (Elsevier); 2003. p. 626-7.
[21] Varma BRR, Nayak RP. Acute Gingival Infections. In: Varma BRR, Nayak RP. *Clinical Periodontology*. Revised ed. New Delhi (India): Arya Publishing House; 2005. p. 156.
[22] Pogrel MA. Complications of Third Molar Surgery. In: Kaban LB, Pogrel MA, Perrott DH. *Complications in Oral and Maxillofacial Surgery*. Philadelphia: Saunders (Elsevier); 1997. p. 60.

In: A Window on Surgery and Orthodontics
Editor: Giuseppe Alessandro Scardina

ISBN: 978-1-62808-948-6

Chapter III

Loop Position in Anterior Retraction Arch Wire and Its Effects on the Produced Forces: 3D Analysis Using Finite Element Method

Allahyar Geramy[1*], Jean Marc Retrouvey[2], Majid Shalchi[1] and Hasan Salehi[3]
[1]Orthodontics Department
Tehran University of Medical Sciences (TUMS), Iran
[2]Orthodontic Division, McGill University, Canada
[3]Orthodontist

Reducing an increased overjet is an acceptable reason to start an orthodontic treatment to improve esthetics and function of the teeth. Different techniques and disciplines have explained anterior retraction according to their goals and appliance designs. One to ten percent of Caucasian orthodontic patients have one or two missing lateral incisors. [1] Achieving esthetic, functional and long-term stable results in orthodontic treatment of these patients require controlled crown and root movements of remaining teeth.

Ever since the Andrews' [2] straight-wire appliance was introduced commercially, many new bracket prescriptions and techniques have been developed and modified as treatment mechanics progress. These developments all move toward one ultimate goal which is to create a force system that can work efficiently and shorten the orthodontic treatment period [3, 4] Until now detailed investigations concerning the effect of wire material or cross-section, [5-9] loop size or configuration, [5, 10-16] loop positioning in segmented arch techniques [17-18], gable bends [7, 14, 18-22], amount of activation or force magnitude, [21]

* Corresponding Author: Dr Allahyar Geramy, Orthodontics Department, School of Dental Medicine, Tehran University of Medical Sciences, North Kargar St. Tehran-IRAN. E-mail: gueramya@tums.ac.ir.

attachment/ligation methods, [22] and en masse or two-step retraction techniques on teeth movements have been conducted [23].

Distance between the applied force and the center of resistance (CRes) of a tooth or a dental segment have a critical influence on tooth movement. The position of CRes in anterior dental segment differs when one or two lateral incisors are missing, therefore the amount and even type of force acting on central incisors, canines, and moment/force ratio (M/F) may be different in such cases. Improper use of closing orthodontic loops may cause adverse results, such as uncontrolled uprighting of the anterior teeth, root resorption, lengthening and complicating treatment or even causing irreversible damage to treatment outcomes.

The main difference between the loop function in a segmented arch technique and a continuous one is a bi-plane expectation in their function which is their new role in a plane perpendicular to theirs. Loops are considered to act in the direction of pulling their legs apart (in open ones) when used to bring teeth together in a segmented arch technique but incorporating a loop in the anterior retraction arch wire brings a bi-plane function to the loop, "A bi-axial activation/deactivation process". Anterior retraction is a process containing two mutually related movements which are expected to be done simultaneously: retracting the anterior teeth (an antero-posterior movement) and providing a good canines-lateral incisor contact (a medio-lateral movement).

Finite element method (FEM) is a numerical analysis to find approximate solutions which is the only possible method in complex structure/problems. This method is new in medical sciences and has proven its efficiencies in different fields. Three-dimensional FEM is a powerful tool used to examine complex mechanical behaviors of dental structures. Evidences are enough to prove its efficiency in analyzing dental biomechanical problems. [24-29].

The main goals of this study were to analyze the effects of anterior retraction loop position on the forces produced and applied on canine, anterior, and posterior teeth. The second goal was to consider the situation in a more generalized view of presence and absence of the lateral incisor while retracting the anterior teeth.

Materials and Methods

Four 3D finite element models were designed of an anterior retraction arch wire with L-loop and included four anterior brackets and the lingual walls of both canine brackets slot for the first stage of the study. (Figure 1a-d) The only difference between models was in the loop position which varied between a near position to the lateral incisor, a normal position, a far position from the lateral incisor, and a special situation when lateral incisors were missing. In the second stage, an L-loop was designed separately. Solid Works 2006 (300 Baker Ave. Concord, Massachusetts 01742, USA) was selected for the modeling phase. The next phase was to transfer the models for calculation to the ANSYS Workbench Ver. 11. 0 (ANSYS Inc. Soutpointe, 275 Technology drive, Cononsburg PA 15317, USA). The mechanical properties of the Stainless Steel were applied using material properties library of the ANSYS Workbench. Models were meshed with 68465 nodes; 28694 10-node-quadratic tetrahedron body elements, 3624 contact elements. (Figure 2)

The boundary condition consisted of fixing the bracket bases and avoiding the arch wire distal to the loops from vertical displacements. Arch wire ends were displaced distally 1 mm and medially 0. 1 mm on each side simulating the activation regarding the arch wire form. Force reactions were assessed in the anterior brackets available in an antero-posterior direction, in canine bracket slot in a medio-lateral direction, and in the distal end of the arch wire in an antero-posterior direction.

The first evaluation was to find the effects of these loops positions on the anterior retraction force on the incisors. The second assessment showed the effects on the canine and the last one tried to assess the protrusive force acting on the terminal molars.

In the second stage, a loop was activated with varying directions (angles) to the loop plane. These angles were 0, 10, 20, 30, 45 degrees to the loop plane. The activation was 1 mm in all stages but decomposed in two planes.

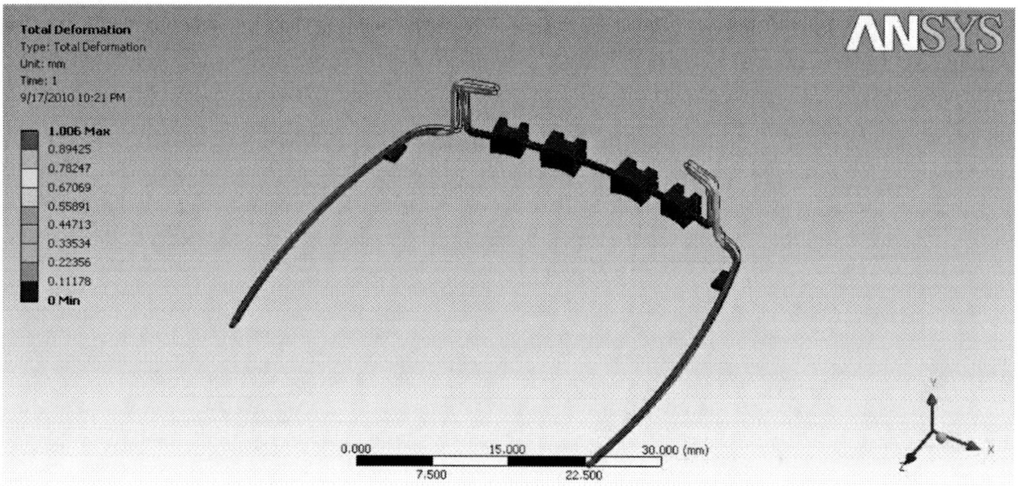

Figure 1a. Loop in normal position.

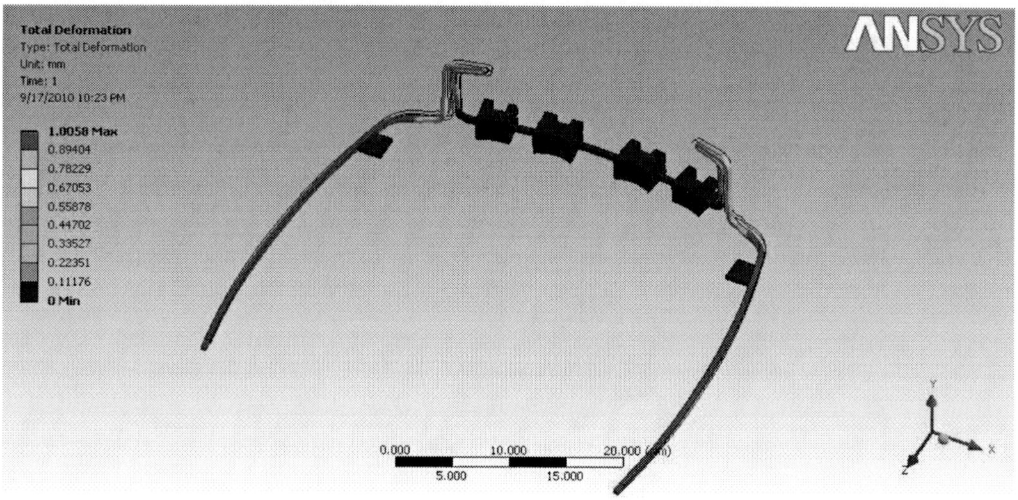

Figure 1b. Loop near to the lateral incisor.

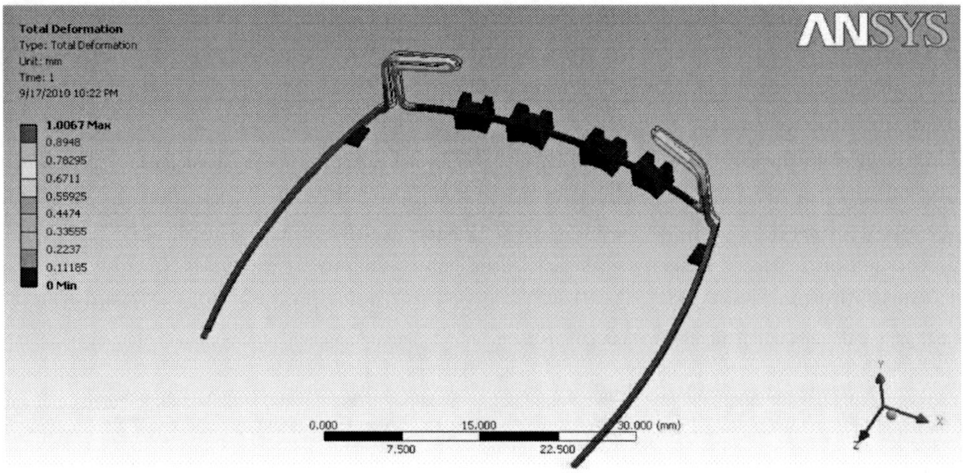

Figure 1c. Loop far away from the lateral incisor.

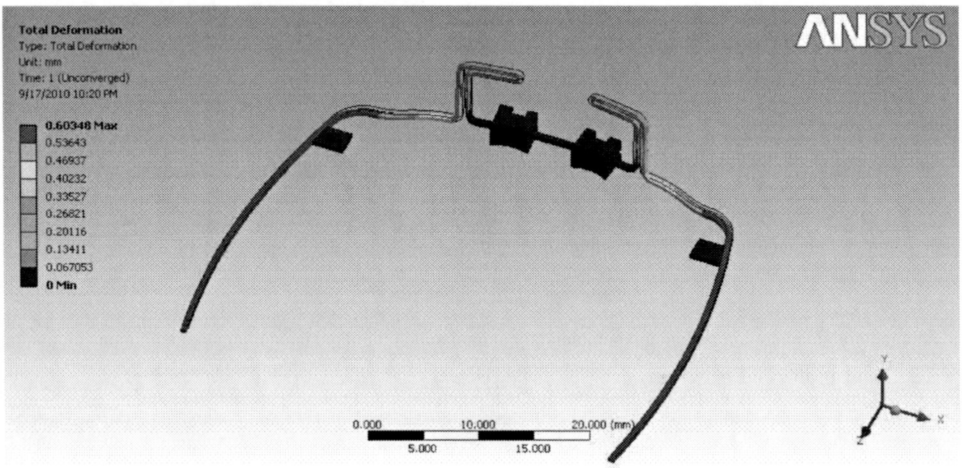

Figure 1d. Loop formed in the lateral incisor position.

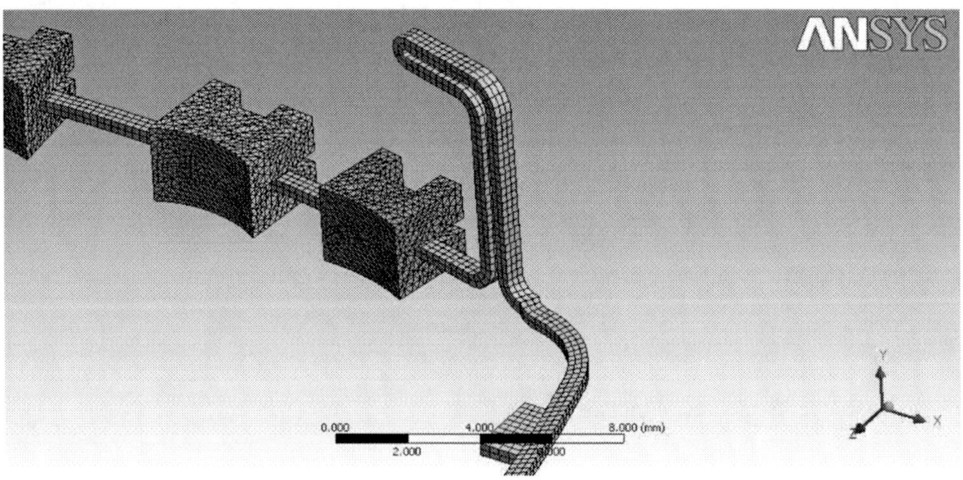

Figure 2. The meshed model in a close view.

Results

The numeric findings were divided into two parts:

The first group of findings was related to the loop positions:

1. Mesializing force on terminal molars (Figure 3a-b):
2. This force starts from 2. 95 N in the normal position of the loop and increased to 2. 96 N when the loop shifted towards the lateral incisor. This force decreased to 1. 509 N when the loop was shifted far away from the lateral incisor. In a missing lateral case, if the loop is placed in the missed lateral tooth position, the terminal molar force was reduced to 0. 851 N.
3. Medially directed force on canine (Figure 3a-b):
4. The normal position of loop resulted in a 1. 74 N force which increased to 2. 12 N when the loop was nearer to the lateral incisor. This finding was 0. 87 N when the loop was far from the lateral incisor. In a lateral incisor missing case, the finding was 0. 97 N if the loop was positioned in the missed lateral position.
5. Retraction force on anterior teeth(Figure 3a-b):
6. A small difference in the force recorded was noticed between the normal position of the loop (= 2. 49 N) and the near-to-lateral-position of loop (=2. 45 N). Shifting away from the lateral incisor resulted in a decrease in the retraction force (= 1. 31 N). In the missing lateral case, the finding was 0. 62 N.

The second group of the finding was from the variations in loop activation angles.

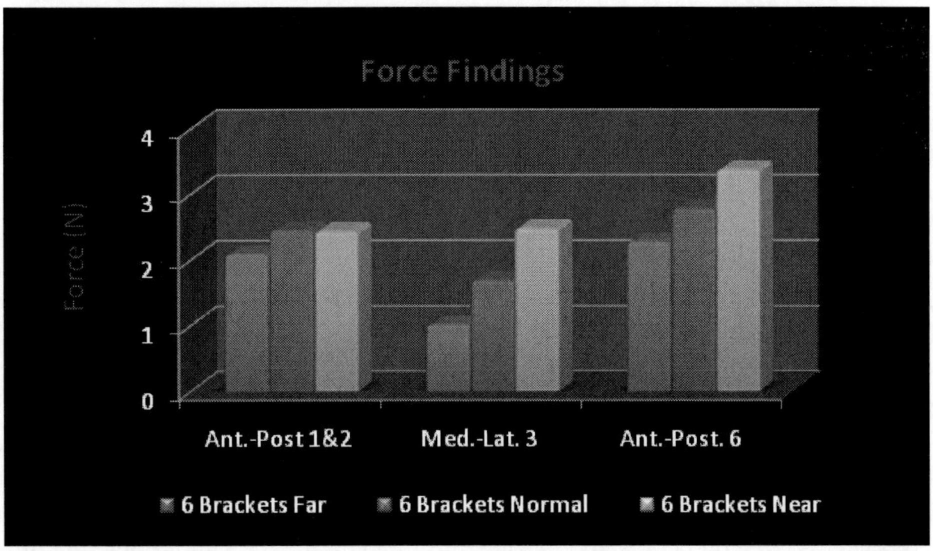

Figure 3a. Different loop position force findings with 6 anterior teeth.

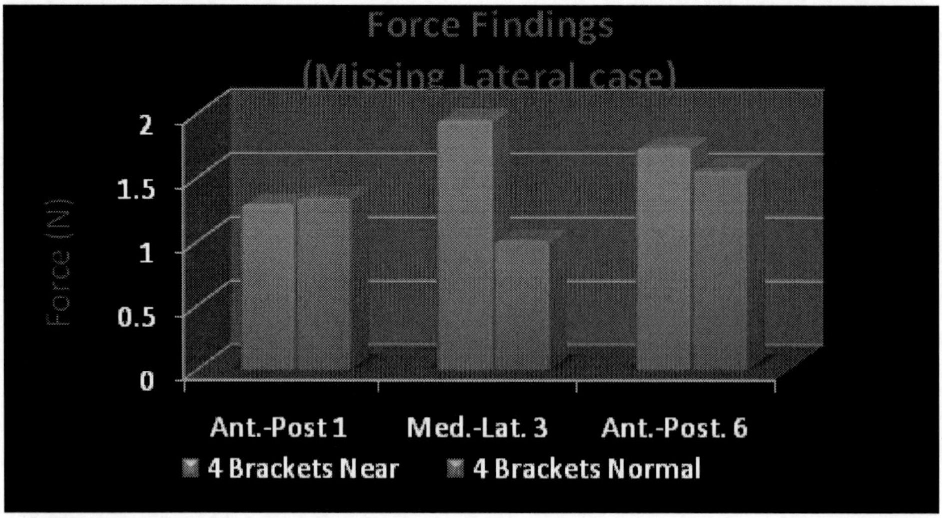

Figure 3b. Different loop position force findings with 4 anterior teeth (missing lateral incisor).

The L- loop force begins with 0. 793 N when activated one millimeter in the loop plane (= 0 deg.) and decreased to 0. 563 N when the force direction was 45 degrees while a new force component was noticed in a plane perpendicular to the loop direction (= 0. 325 N).

In this way, changing the force vector direction from 0 to 45 degrees decreased the force in the direction of the loop while increasing the force vector in a plane perpendicular to the loop one.

Discussion

Loop positions were assessed between the lateral incisor and the canine when the lateral incisors are present or missing. The main question appeared when treating a missing lateral incisor case. The question was" where should we place the loop?" In other words: "does it matter where to place the loop biomechanically?" This question was generalized later as what the effects of loop position on its functions are. In a missing lateral case, it was shown that placing the loop in the missed lateral incisor position or in its normal position (considering the case to have the lateral incisors) does not affect the antero-posterior force on incisors or mesializing force on molars significantly. This position was optimized using the medio-lateral force on canines. Shifting the loop towards the canine decreased the mdeio-lateral force thus making it a suitable loop position to start anterior retraction with an acceptable medio-lateral force on canines and enough wire to be used in consequent stages of retraction between the canines and the loop. In its general form, the loop position was evaluated while retracting four anterior teeth. Shifting from a near position to the lateral incisor to a far position decreased the medio-lateral force on canine and mesializing force on molar. The far position of the loop decreased all force findings. This decrease was more prominent on canine.

The effect of the loop position on the canine force can be explained by focusing on the geometry of the wire between the loop and the canine. This wire geometry, being affected directly by the loop position, connects the anterior part of the arch wire to the posterior one.

In continuous arch wire, forming the anterior retraction loop near to the lateral incisor reinforces two determining factors in the force system present: (these factors are inter-related)

1. The wire curve formed between the canine bracket and the lateral incisor.
2. The difference between the inter-canine width and the inter-lateral bracket width viewing antero-posteriorly.

Figure 5 shows some variations in the geometry of the wire connecting the canine bracket and the loop. Based on the variations shown, forming the curve like the red one dictates a higher medio-lateral force on canine at the start of the retraction than the green one. Activating the arch wire formed like the red one applies a high force on canine due to a sudden change in the arch width thus pulling the legs of the loop away from each other making a rather high force on anterior teeth.

On the contrary, forming the wire segment like the green one, makes it possible to start with a light force on canine (due to a rather straight wire segment anterior to the canine) and the minimum of loop activation along its plane (the loop is activated perpendicular to the loop plane producing a lighter force according to figure 4).

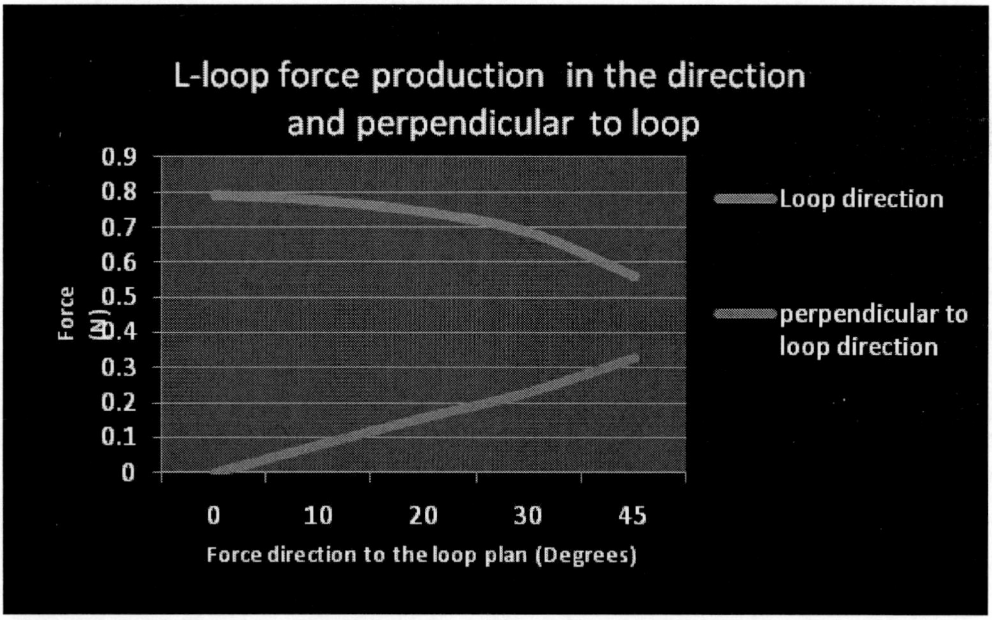

Figure 4. Loop force in two perpendicular plans.

The same is true when retracting central incisors in missing lateral incisor cases. In this situation, the force decline is faster.

It is worth mentioning that a loop when incorporated in a continuous arch wire to retract the anterior teeth is expected to: retract the anterior teeth (an anterio-posterior function); and bring the canines in a good contact with the lateral incisors at the end of the retraction (A medio-lateral function). The loop position in the small distance available between the lateral incisor and canine is responsible for the strategy of dividing the force produced between these two functions during the retraction process.

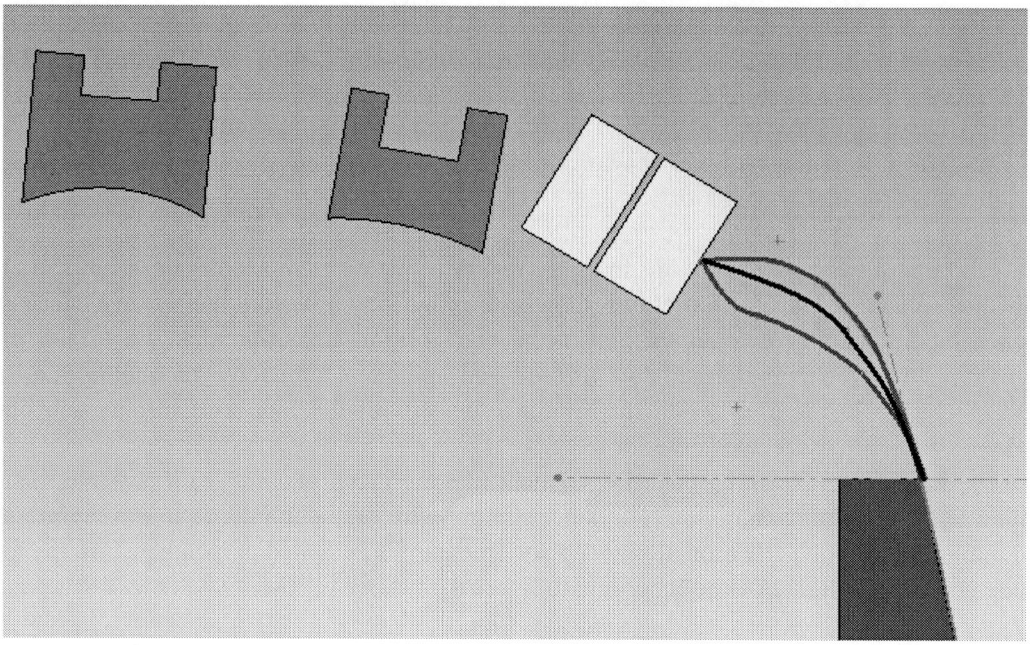

Figure 5. Top view of the right central (red), lateral incisor (red), and canine (blue) bracket. The loop section is shown in yellow. The wire segment between the canine bracket and loop section is shown in three various geometries. (Red, Black, and Green).

Trying to interpret the findings guided to a more generalized concept. Loops are studied by applying force to activate them. What will happen if various force directions are applied? What is the loop behavior under different loop activation directions? In the last stage of this study, a separate loop was activated by a force vector. The force direction to the loop plane was 0 degree (in the loop plane), 10 degrees, 20 degrees, 30 degrees, and 45 degrees. Figure 4 shows the results. Increasing the force angle formed between the force vector and the loop plane decreased the activation force in the plane of the loop and increased the force in a plane perpendicular to the loop. Shifting the loop from a near position to the lateral incisor to a far one, considering the constant position of the canine, increased the angle of force vector to the loop. In this way, the loop force is decreased and increasing its retraction function.

Conclusion

Based on this FEM study it can be concluded that:

1. The loop in the anterior retraction arch wire is suggested to be formed mid-way between the lateral incisor and the canine.
2. In missing lateral incisor cases, the wire is formed so that the tooth/teeth are not missing.
3. A more or less straight wire segment formed mesial to the canine ensures a light force on canine and the anterior teeth. (like the green curve in figure 5).

References

[1] Mattheeuws N, Dermaut L, Martens G. Has hypodontia increased in Caucasians during the 20th century? A meta-analysis. *Eur. J. Orthod.* 2004;26:99-103.

[2] Andrews LF. The six keys to normal occlusion. *Am. J. Orthod.* 1972; 62: 296-309.

[3] Roth RK. Treatment mechanics for the straight wire appliance. In:Graber TM, Swain BF,eds. *Orthodontics: Current Principles and techniques.* St Louis, Mo: CV Mosby;1985: 665-716.

[4] McLughlin RP, Bennet JC. The transition from standard edgewise to preadjusted appliance systems. *J. Clinical Orthod.* 1989;23: 142-53.

[5] Odegaard J, Meling T, Meling E. The effects of loops on the torsional stiffnesses of rectangular wires: an in-vitro study. *Am. J. Orthod. Dentofacial Orthop* 1996;109:496-505.

[6] Menghi C, Planert J, Melsen B. 3-D experimental identification of force systems from orthodontic loops activated for first order corrections. *Angle Orthod* 1999; 69:49-57.

[7] Manhartsberger C, Morton JY, Burstone CJ. Space closure in adult patients using the segmented arch technique. *Angle Orthod* 1989; 59(3):205-10.

[8] Ferreira MA. The wire material and cross-section effect on double delta closing loops regarding load and spring rate magnitude: an in vitro study. *Am. J. Orthod. Dentofacial Orthop.* 1999;115: 275-82.

[9] Rose D, Quick A, Swain M, Herbison P. Moment-to-force characteristics of preactivated nickel-titanium and titanium-molybdenum alloy symmetrical T-loops. *Am. J. Orthod Dentofacial. Orthop.* 2009;135:757-63.

[10] Chaconas SJ, Caputo AA, Hayashi RK. Effects of wire size, loop configuration, and gabling on canine-retraction springs. *Am. J. Orthod.* 1974;65:58-66.

[11] Lipsett AW, Faulkner MG, el-Rayes K. Large deformation analysis of orthodontic appliances. *J. Biomech. Eng.* 1990;112:29-37.

[12] Siatkowski RE. Continuous arch wire closing loop design, optimization, and verification. *Part I. Am. J. Orthod DentofacialOrthop.* 1997;112:393-402.

[13] Chen J, Chen K, Katona TR, Baldwin JJ, Arbuckle GR. Nonlinear large deformation FE analysis of orthodontic springs. *Biomed. Mater. Eng.* 1997;7:99-110.

[14] Sander FG. Biomechanical investigation of the hybrid retraction spring. *J. Orofac Orthop.* 2000;61(5):341-51.

[15] Raboud D, Faulkner G, Lipsett B, Haberstock D. Three dimensional force systems from vertically activated orthodontic loops. *Am. J. Orthod. Dentofacial. Orthop* 2001;119:21-9.

[16] Blaya MB, Westphalen GH, Guimaraes MB, Hirakata LM. Evaluation of tensile strength of different configurations of orthodontic retraction loops for obtaining optimized forces. *Stomatologija* 2009;11:66-69.

[17] Kuhlberg AJ, Burstone CJ. T-loop position and anchorage control. *Am. J. Orthod Dentofacial Orthop.* 1997;112: 12-8.

[18] Mazza D, Mazza M. Specialized spring design in segmented edgewise orthodontics: further verification of dedicated software. *Angle Orthod* 2000;70: 52-62.

[19] Katona TR, Le YP, Chen J. The effects of first- and second-order gable bends on forces and moments generated by triangular loops. *Am. J. Orthod. Dentofacial Orthop* 2006;129:54-9.

[20] Martins RP, Buschang PH, Martins LP, Gandini LG. Optimizing the design of preactivated titanium T-loop springs with loop software. *Am. J. Orthod. Dentofacial Orthop*. 2008;134:161-6.

[21] Ren Y, Maltha J C, Kuijpers-Jagtman AM. Optimum force magnitude for orthodontic tooth movement: a systematic literature review. *Angle Orthod* 2003. 73:86–92.

[22] Koenig HA, Burstone CJ. Force systems from an ideal arch:large deflection considerations. *Angle Orthod* 1989;59: 11-6.

[23] Heo W, Nahm DS, Baek SH. En masse retraction and two-step retraction of maxillary anterior teeth in adult class I women. *Angle Orthod* 2007; 77(6):973-8.

[24] Geramy A. Alveolar bone resorption and the center of resistance modification: 3D analysis by means of the F. E. M. *Am. J. Orthod Dentofacial Orthop. 2000;* 117: 399-405.

[25] Geramy A. Stresses around a mini screw. 3D analysis with the finite element method (FEM). *Aust. Orthod. J.* 2009; 25(2): 104-9.

[26] Geramy A. Optimization of unilateral overjet management: 3D analysis using finite element method. *The Angle Orthod* 2002; 75(6):585-92.

[27] Geramy A, Morgano S. Finite element analysis of three designs of an implant-supported molar crown. *J. Prosthetic Dent.* 2004; 92:434-40.

[28] Geramy A, Ghadirian H. Comparison of methods used to correct a lingually tilted mandibular molar: 3-D analysis using the finite element method (FEM). *Aust . Orthod J.* 2008; 24:96-101.

[29] Geramy A, Faghihi Sh. Secondary trauma from occlusion: 3D analysis using finite element method. *Quintessence Intl.* 2004; 35:835-43.

In: A Window on Surgery and Orthodontics
Editor: Giuseppe Alessandro Scardina
ISBN: 978-1-62808-948-6

Chapter IV

Comparative Evaluation of Subepithelial Connective Tissue Graft and Acellular Dermal Matrix Graft in the Treatment of Gingival Recession – A Case Series

Nikesh N. Moolya**[*1]**, Swati B. Setty**[2]**,
***Srinath Thakur**[2]** and S. Ravindra**[3]*
[1]Department of Periodontics,
Padmashree Dr. D. Y. Patil Dental College and Hospital, Nerul,
Navi Mumbai, India
[2]Department of Periodontics, SDM College of Dental Sciences and Hospital,
Dharwad, Karnataka, India
[3]Department of Periodontics, Hassan Dental College, Karnataka, India

Abstract

Aims: To clinically evaluate and compare efficacy of acellular dermal matrix allograft and sub epithelial connective tissue graft in the treatment of gingival recession.

Methods: A randomized clinical trial was conducted where twenty eight patients presenting gingival recession ≤ 4 mm were treated for recession coverage and received either acellular dermal matrix (ADM) or sub epithelial connective tissue (CTG). Prior to and at the end of 3, 6 and 9 months the parameters assessed were: plaque index (PI), gingival index (GI), probing depth(PD), recession depth(RD), relative attachment level(RAL) and width of keratinized tissue(KT). The percentage of root coverage was also calculated and data were statistically analyzed by student's paired t test.

[*] Address for correspondence: Dr. Nikesh N. Moolya, Department of Periodontics, Padmashree Dr. D. Y. Patil Dental College and Hospital, Nerul, Navi Mumbai, Maharashtra, India. E-mail: drmoolya@gmail.com.

Results: Both groups yielded improvements in PI, GI, RD decrease, gain in RAL and gain in width of keratinized tissue. The root coverage was 56. 32 % for ADM group and 72. 78 % for CTG group respectively. CTG group produced a greater increase in all the evaluated parameters compared to ADM group.

Conclusion: The present data appeared to indicate that subepithelial connective tissue graft group showed better clinical improvements than acellular dermal matrix graft group in all the parameters assessed.

Keywords: Acellular dermal matrix, connective tissue, randomized clinical trial, recession, keratinized tissue

Introduction

In the current practice of periodontics, clinicians are faced with the challenge of not only addressing biological and functional problems present in the periodontium, but also providing a periodontal therapy that result in acceptable esthetics. The exposure of root surfaces due to gingival recession can pose a multitude of problems like hypersensitivity, root surface caries along with a massive esthetic deficiency. A wide variety of periodontal plastic surgical procedures have thus been described to cover denuded root surfaces and to correct other mucogingival problems [1, 2, 3]. Roccuzo et al. in their systematic review mentioned that periodontal plastic surgery was effective in reducing gingival recession with a concomitant improvement in attachment levels [4]. Keeping these objectives in mind, the search for the perfect root coverage technique has taken many differing approaches. It has been demonstrated that the underlying connective tissues had a direct bearing on the type of epithelium that is superimposed upon it [5]. It was shown that a significant increase in attached gingiva can be achieved by grafting gingival connective tissue alone [6]. Langer and Langer described the "Sub Epithelial Connective tissue graft" technique in detail for covering gingival recessions on both single and multiple adjacent teeth [7]. By incorporating the advantages of the pedicle graft such as the double blood supply from the overlying flap and the periosteal connective tissue bed coupled with the genetic potential of the connective tissue from the palate, it was possible to maximize the graft survival and also provided excellent esthetics. Although auto grafts have proven predictable they are not without few drawbacks. The donor tissue is usually harvested from the hard palate which necessitates an additional surgical procedure on the patient. The drawbacks inherent with auto grafts have instigated a search for alternate approaches.

It has been demonstrated that allogenic freeze-dried skin graft was clinically acceptable as grafts for the treatment of mucogingival problems. An "Acellular Dermal Graft"has been developed with significant advantages over the previous freeze dried skin allografts. The allograft is obtained from a human donor skin tissue process that removes its cell components while preserving the remaining bioactive components and the extra cellular matrix which is subsequently freeze dried. It exhibits undamaged collagen and elastin matrices that function as a scaffold to allow ingrowth by host tissues. Thus the integrity of the extra-cellular matrix is maintained which is responsible for inflammatory response associated with the earlier available freeze-dried skin allografts. These unique characteristics make the acellular dermal matrix allograft completely biocompatible and safe [8-15].

The aim of the present study was to evaluate in vivo the efficacy of Acellular Dermal Matrix Allograft (ADM) and Sub epithelial Connective tissue Graft (CTG) as a root coverage material and also to compare the clinical results of Acellular Dermal Matrix with Sub epithelial Connective tissue graft in treatment of gingival recession.

Material and Methods

Twenty eight systemically healthy patients (15 males, 13 females) in good gingival health with Miller's Grade I and Grade II recession belonging to age group of 29-51(mean age 34. 5±2) years were selected for the chapter. This was a randomized single blinded clinical trial and patients with esthetic concerns and hypersensitivity were selected for the chapter. Patients with root surface restorations on surgical sites and smokers were excluded from the chapter. Patients were randomly divided into 2 groups to receive either Sub epithelial Connective tissue graft or Acellular Dermal Matrix graft (Alloderm Regenerative Matrix, Life Cell, BioHorizons, USA) and followed up for a period of 9 months. The informed consent regarding the benefits and protocol of the study was obtained from all the patients. The clinical parameters like plaque index. (PI) [16], gingival index (GI) [17], probingdepth (PD), recession depth. (RD), relative attachment level (RAL), width of keratinized tissue (KT) and percentage of root coverage (RC) [18] were assessed at baseline, 3, 6 and 9 months. All the measurements were made with a UNC-15 probe (Hu-friedy, USA). The selected sites were randomly allocated as

1. ADM group (Figure 1)
2. CTG group (Figure 2)

All the patients underwent comprehensive periodontal treatment that included detailed oral hygiene instructions, scaling, root planning and occlusal adjustment if necessary. Acrylic stents were made for the treatment sites to increase precision and reproducibility of measurements.

Surgical Technique

The surgical area in the ADM group was prepared with adequate anesthesia using 2% Lignocaine HCI containing 1:80,000 epinephrine. The incision design introduced by Zucchelli avoiding vertical incisions was used throughout the chapter [19]. Full thickness mucoperiosteal flap reflection was extended to 3 mm apical to the alveolar bone crest using a periosteal elevator, followed by split thickness flap reflection. Full thickness flap dissection was extended mesially, distally and apically to facilitate adequate mobility and coronal positioning of the flap without tension using a number 15 Bard Parker blade (Aspen Surgical Products, USA) (Figure 1a). The root was thoroughly planed and any convexities of the root were reduced. The exposed root surface was conditioned with 24% EDTA (PrefGel, Straumann Biologics Division, Waltham, MA, USA) for 2 minutes to remove the smear layer and thoroughly rinsed with saline for 30 seconds [20]. It was rehydrated by submerging in 50 cc of saline at 37 degree celsius sterile normal saline for 30 minutes. After peeling the backing and once the tissue was fully rehydrated, ADM was placed under the flap. ADM was oriented so that the basement membrane side was placed adjacent to the defect [21, 22, 23]. Firm pressure was applied on the graft with a sterile moist gauze pack for 3 to 5 minutes to help the graft adapt and adhere to the recipient wound bed. It was secured to the wound bed with 5-0 Polyglactin vicryl sutures (Ethicon, Inc. Somerville, New Jersey) (Figure 1b). The CTG was harvested from the palate following a trap door flap design [24]. A number 15 Bard Parker blade was used to make a partial thickness horizontal incision with a bevel about 3 mm apical to the gingival margin of the first premolar extending towards first molar (Figure 2a). Two vertical incisions were made mesiodistally. Tissue forceps was used to lift the prepared palatal edge. It was reflected towards the centre of the palate and the underlying connective tissue was exposed. An incision perpendicular to the bone was made around the centre of the palate and the underlying connective tissue was exposed.

An incision perpendicular to the bone was made around the edge of the connective tissue facilitating its reflection from bone. A small periosteal elevator and Kirkland knife were used to reflect the connective tissue and harvest it. The harvested CTG was placed on the denuded root and stabilized with 5-0 polyglactin vicryl sutures (Ethicon, Inc., Somerville, New Jersey). Both ADM and CTG surgical sites were covered by periodontal dressing (Coe-Pak, Alsip, GC, IL, USA) for two weeks with replacing at one week interval.

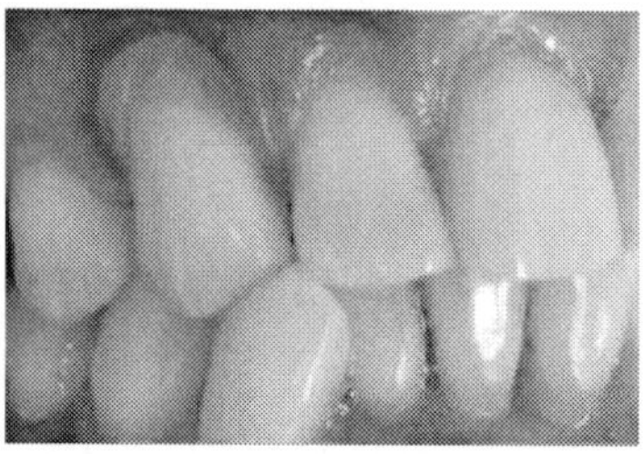

Figure 1. Preoperative ADM group.

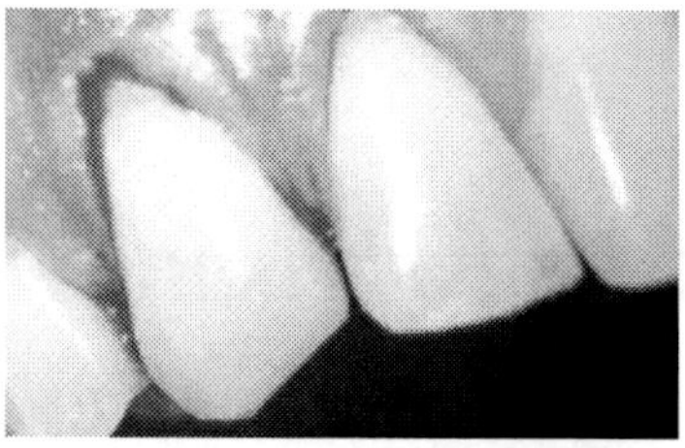

Figure 1a. Incision and Envelope technique.

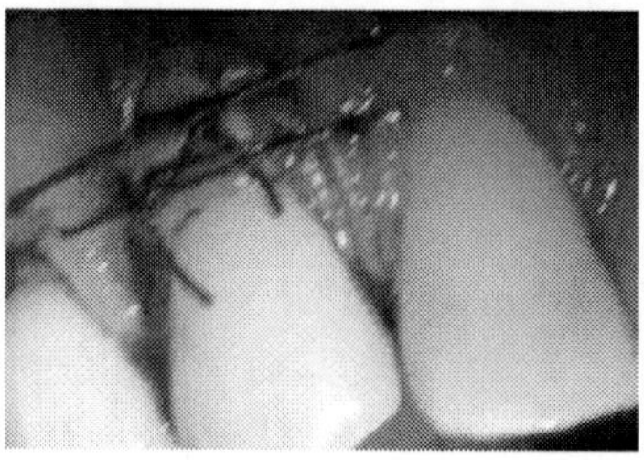

Figure 1b. Placement of ADM on the recipient site and stabilization with 5-0 vicryl sutures.

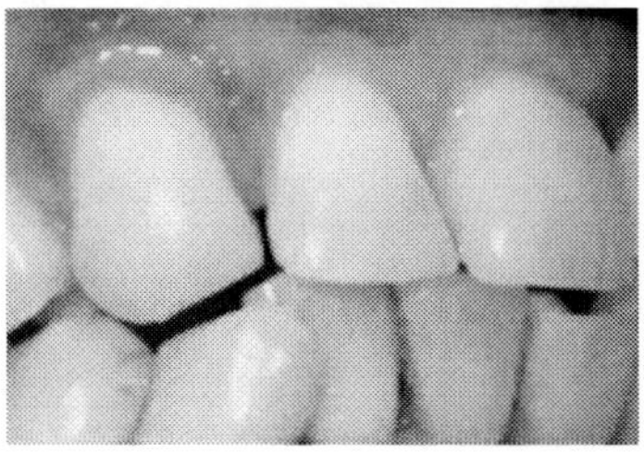

Figure 1c. Postoperative 3 months.

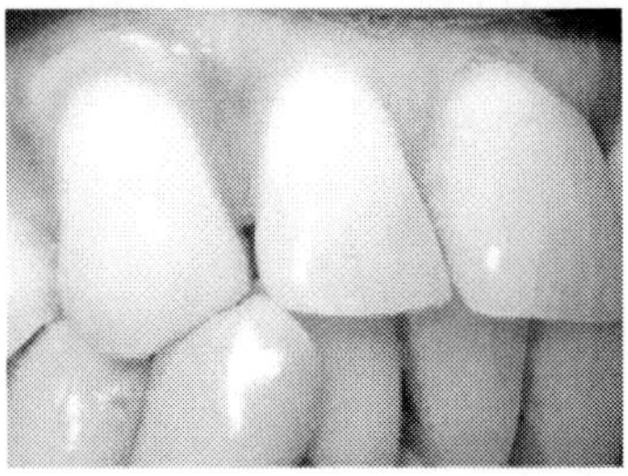

Figure 1d. Postoperative 9 months.

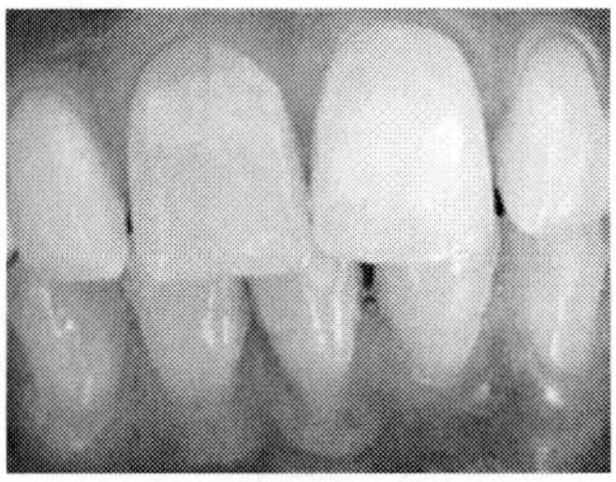

Figure 2. Preoperative CTG group.

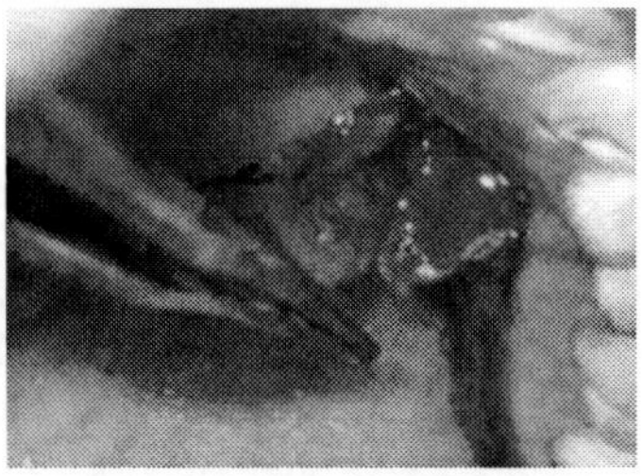

Figure 2a. Harvesting of subepithelial connective tissue graft from palate.

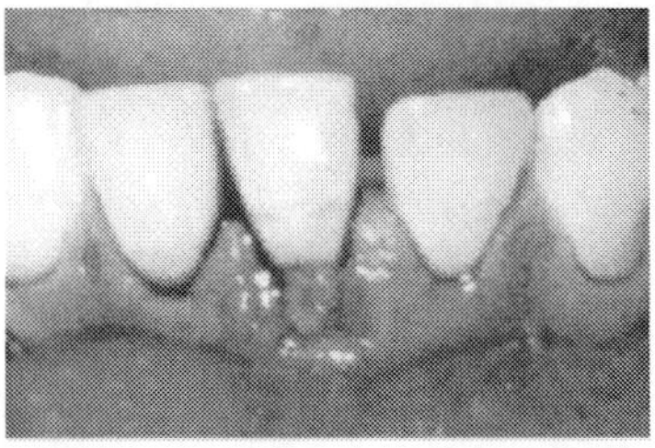

Figure 2b. Placement of CTG on recipient site.

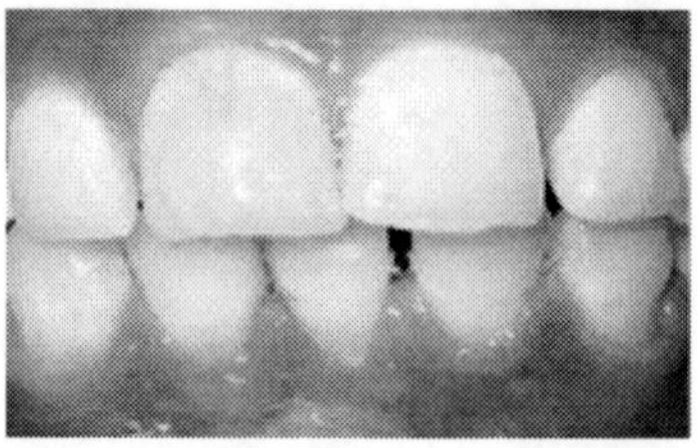

Figure 2c. Postoperative 3 months.

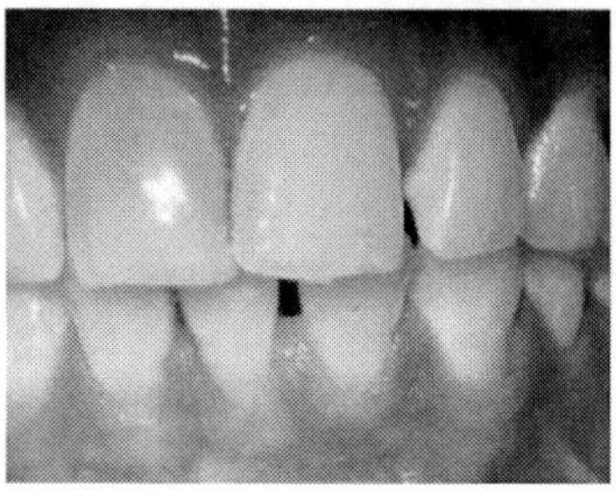

Figure 2d. Postoperative 9 months.

Post Surgical Care

The post-surgical care in both groups follows previous studies from Cueva and Shin [25, 26]. Briefly, gentle ice pack application was used immediately after surgery on a 20 minute intermittent basis for the first 24 hours at both CTG and ADM sites. All patients were advised to use cotton tipped applicators saturated with chlorhexidine gluconate 0. 12% on the surgical sites for 4 weeks, and avoid trauma to the surgical sites. Amoxicillin 500 mg three-times-a-day for 5 days was prescribed and analgesics were prescribed as needed to prevent any incidence of postoperative infection and bacteremia. The sutures were removed at 14 days. The patients were instructed to resume gentle mechanical tooth brushing after 15 days on the treated sites. Both ADM Group and CTG Group sites were evaluated postoperatively 3rd, 6th and 9th month after surgery. On each visit, the area was checked for meticulous plaque control but no sub gingival instrumentation was performed, Clinical measurements were recorded and mean percentage of coverage calculated both for ADM Group and CTG Group sites.

Statistical Analysis

The clinical data obtained were fed into the computer using Microsoft Excel 2000 package and statistical analysis was carried out. The data i. e. plaque index, gingival index, probing depth, recession depth, relative attachment level, and width of keratinized tissue at baseline and at end of three, six and nine months after surgery was first collected. Following this the data was subjected to statistical analysis using Student's paired t test. Data analysis was performed using SPSS (version 11) software.

Results

Uneventful healing was observed with all the ADM and CTG grafts. (Figure 1c, 1d, 2c, 2d). Complete maturation and stability of the tissue was obtained at 3 months and remained stable till 9 months. Comparative evaluation of ADM group and CTG group showed a reduction in mean plaque values from 0. 622 mm to 0. 492 in ADM group and 0. 708 to 0. 369 mm in CTG group 9 months postoperatively (Table 1).

Table 1. Comparison of ADM and CTG group

		ADM Group		CTG Group				
		Mean	Std. Dev.	Mean	Std. Dev.	t-value	P-value	Signi.
Plaque	Preoperative	0. 6220	0. 1978	0. 7080	0. 1677	-1. 0486	0. 3082	NS
	3 months	0. 4180	0. 1221	0. 4840	0. 1151	-1. 2438	0. 2295	NS
	6 months	0. 4330	0. 1029	0. 3950	0. 1120	0. 7903	0. 4396	NS
	9 months	0. 4920	0. 1312	0. 3690	0. 0684	2. 6287	0. 0170	S
Gingival index	Preoperative	0. 7230	0. 4418	0. 5030	0. 2246	1. 4037	0. 1774	NS
	3 months	0. 2993	0. 2687	0. 3030	0. 1175	-0. 0399	0. 9686	NS
	6 months	0. 3060	0. 3911	0. 2460	0. 1071	0. 4679	0. 6454	NS
	9 months	0. 1372	0. 1212	0. 2470	0. 0909	-2. 2917	0. 0342	S
Probing depth	Preoperative	1. 0000	0. 0000	1. 1000	0. 3162	-1. 0000	0. 3306	NS
	3 months	0. 8500	0. 2415	0. 8000	0. 2582	0. 4472	0. 6601	NS
	6 months	0. 8500	0. 2415	0. 8000	0. 2582	0. 4472	0. 6601	NS
	9 months	0. 8500	0. 2415	0. 8000	0. 2582	0. 4472	0. 6601	NS
Recession depth	Preoperative	3. 1000	0. 7379	3. 3000	0. 5869	-0. 6708	0. 5109	NS
	3 months	1. 5000	0. 6667	1. 0500	0. 4378	1. 7842	0. 0913	NS
	6 months	1. 5000	0. 6667	1. 0000	0. 4082	2. 0226	0. 0582	NS
	9 months	1. 3000	0. 6749	0. 9000	0. 3944	1. 6181	0. 1230	NS
Relative Attachment level	Preoperative	10. 7500	1. 3591	10. 8500	1. 8567	-0. 1374	0. 8922	NS
	3 months	8. 9500	1. 7709	8. 2500	1. 8447	0. 8657	0. 3981	NS
	6 months	8. 8500	1. 6675	8. 2000	1. 8439	0. 8268	0. 4192	NS
	9 months	8. 7000	1. 8288	8. 1000	1. 7920	0. 7410	0. 4682	NS
Width of Keratinized tissue	Preoperative	2. 8000	0. 3496	2. 7500	0. 4859	0. 2641	0. 7947	NS
	3 months	4. 3500	0. 7091	4. 9500	0. 5986	-2. 0447	0. 0558	NS
	6 months	4. 3500	0. 7091	5. 0000	0. 6667	-2. 1120	0. 0489	S
	9 months	4. 5500	0. 8317	5. 1000	0. 7746	-1. 5303	0. 1433	NS
Root coverage		56. 3260	27. 3963	72. 7800	10. 7263	-1. 7685	0. 0939	NS

*** P<0. 001 – Significant(S). *** P>0. 001 - Not Significant(NS).

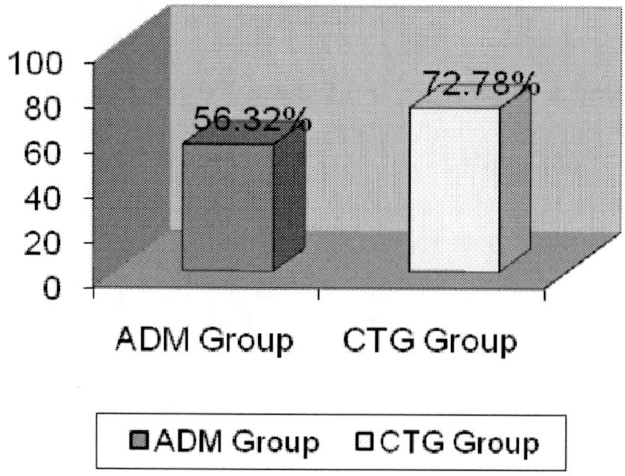

Table 2. Percentage of root coverage.

Comparison between the two groups was statistically significant with greater reduction in CTG group at a p-value of 0. 0170 (*** P<0. 001,S) (Table 1).

Gingival index values in ADM group reduced from 0. 723 mm to 0. 137 and 0. 503 to 0. 247 mm in CTG group 9 months postoperatively (Table 1). Comparison between the two groups was statistically significant with greater reduction in CTG group at a p-value of 0. 0342 (*** P<0. 001,S) (Table 1).

Comparative evaluation of ADM group and CTG group showed a reduction in mean probing pocket depth from 1mm to 0. 85 in ADM group and 1. 1 to 0. 8 mm in CTG group 9 months postoperatively (Table 1) though comparison between the two groups was not statistically significant at a p-valueof 0. 66 (*** P>0. 001, NS)(Table 1). Comparative evaluation of ADM group and CTG group showed a reduction in mean recession depth from 3. 1 mm to 1. 3 in ADM group and 3. 3 to 0. 9 mm in CTG group 9 months postoperatively (Table 1).

Comparison between the two groups was not statistically significant with greater reduction in CTG group at a p-value of 0. 123(*** P<0. 001, S) (Table 1). The mean difference in ADM group was 1. 8 mm and the mean difference in CTG group was 2. 4 mm. Comparative evaluation of ADM group and CTG group showed a reduction in relative attachment level from 10. 75 mm to 8. 7 in ADM group and 10. 85 mm to 8. 7mm in CTG group 9 months postoperatively (Table 1).

Comparison between the two groups was not statistically significant with greater reduction in CTG group at a p-value of 0. 4682 (*** P<0. 001, S) (Table 1). The mean difference in ADM group was 2. 05 mm and the mean difference in CTG group was 2. 75 mm. Comparative evaluation between ADM group and CTG group showed an increase in width of keratinized tissue from 2. 8 to 4. 5 in Group A and 2. 75 to 5. 1 mm in CTG group 9 months postoperatively (Table 1).

The mean increase in width of keratinized tissue was 1. 75 mm in ADM group while the mean increase in width of keratinized tissue was more in CTG Group at 2. 35 mm. The comparison between the groups was not statistically significant (Table 1). The percentage of root coverage with ADM was 56. 32 %. and with CTG was 72. 78 % 9 months postoperatively (Table 2).

Discussion

The findings of this randomized single blinded trial showed a statistically significant reduction in plaque index, gingival index, recession depth, relative attachment level and significant increase in width of keratinized tissue in both ADM group and CTG group. The mean plaque index and gingival index showed a reduction in values in both ADM group and CTG group. These values may be attributed to the improved oral hygiene at recall visits and regular reinforcements. Mean probing depth did not show any statistical significant changes at 3, 6 and 9 months. This result was expected because baseline probing depth in all patients was compatible with a condition of gingival health. The results obtained in this chapter was also consistent with the chapter done by Tal et al. where clinically it was difficult to penetrate the sulcus with a probe post operatively [27]. The mean recession depth decreased from 3. 1 mm to 1. 3 mm in ADM group and 3. 3 mm to 0. 9 mm in CTG group. The decrease in CTG was more than ADM but a comparison between the groups was not statistically significant. These values were comparable to the chapter by Rahmani et al. where they found a reduction in recession depth of 3. 5 mm to1. 85 mm in ADM group and reduction of 3. 1 mm to 1. 4 mm in CTG group [28]. Few subjects in the chapter did show a reduction of 0. 1-0. 2 mm in recession depth between the 3rd and 9th month post operatively. This amount of root coverage could be attributed to creeping attachment. Borghetti and Gardella suggested any increase in attachment after 1 month of healing should be considered creeping attachment [29]. The gain in relative attachment level was 2. 05 mm in ADM group and 2. 75 in CTG group. In a similar chapter by Rahmani et al. comparing CTG and ADM they found a gain in attachment levels of 2. 75 mm and 2. 05 mm in ADM and CTG respectively [28]. These clinical findings are compatible with a healthy attachment. The mean increase in width of keratinized tissue was 1. 75 mm in ADM group while the gain was more in CTG group at 2. 35 mm. In a comparative study on the effectiveness of ADM to increase attached gingiva, Wei et al. reported that ADM produced a lesser extent of attached tissue in comparison with CTG [30]. These authors ascribed this result to the considerable shrinkage of ADM during the healing stage. ADM is a non vital connective tissue. It is also conceivable that viability of connective tissue may be essential for a graft to fully express the capability of inducing keratinization of the overlaying epithelium [24]. However other authors [9] do not agree with this hypothesis. ADM acts as a scaffold for cells from the surrounding tissues and the original non vital graft is degraded and completely replaced by host cells. Considering that only the cells from the periodontal ligament and gingival connective tissue are capable of inducing the development of a keratinized epithelium, the inductive properties of ADM grafts will depend on the colonization of the nonvital graft by host cell deriving from these tissues capable of inducing keratinization. ADM taken from keratinized tissue could present the same inductionability. On the other hand it is known that epithelialization of CTG available from keratinized sites result in keratinized epithelium via an induction mechanism [5]. The mean root coverage obtained with CTG was 72. 78% and with the ADM root coverage was 56. 32%. These results compare favorably with percentage of root covered as reported by Bouchard et al. (69%) [31] and Rahmani (65. 2%) [28] but less favorably with results of Harris RJ (87%) [32]. Envelope technique was used for the treatment of all single isolated recessions in this study in order to facilitate early healing, good color matching, no incision or suture marks [19]. Raetzke suggested that covering the graft with flap provides enough blood supply to nourish the uncovered portion of the graft over the denuded root [33]. High flap tension lowers recession coverage as put forth by Pini Prato [34]. Flap retraction may result in loss of exposed graft resulting in incomplete root coverage. That may be one of the reasons for the low percentage of root coverage in both ADM and CTG groups in this chapter. In this study an increased gingival margin thickness was observed with use of both ADM and CTG groups. This was a clinical impression and was not quantitated. This merits further study to determine the effect of marginal thickness in preventing future recession. Henderson et al. hypothesized that marginal tissue thickness maybe a more critical determinant of future recession than width of keratinized tissue [35]. A systematic review by Wang also suggested that a positive association exists between weighted flap thickness and mean and complete root coverage [36]. Thus mean root coverage in both the groups does imply that both surgical procedures have definite therapeutic utility in the clinical practice. The results showed that both periodontal plastic surgical treatments significantly improved the clinical parameters evaluated in this study from baseline to 9 months. One of the limitations of this chapter was that the recession width was not assessed which may be a critical factor in determining the amount of root coverage. Another limitation would be a small sample size and lack of long term evaluation in both the groups. A subjective evaluation of the two groups was not done but the clinical impression gave better results for use of sub epithelial connective tissue grafts. Long term evaluation will thus go a long way in substantiating the efficacy and also the stability of Acellular Dermal Matrix graft as a coveted alternative for recession cases when viewed on par with the current "Gold standard" namely Sub epithelial Connective tissue grafts [37]. Further research is needed to improve methods of measurement of exposed root surface in order to assess long term success of such procedures.

Conclusion

The present data appeared to indicate that Subepithelial Connective tissue graft group showed better clinical improvements than Acellular Dermal Matrix graft group in all the parameters assessed. Clinical evaluation was suggestive of the fact that Acellular Dermal Matrix graft did not elicit any untoward host response. Acellular Dermal Matrix graft can act as an effective substitute for Sub epithelial Connective tissue graft in the treatment of gingival recession. Both, Sub epithelial Connective tissue graft and Acellular Dermal Matrix graft were useful and predictable surgical techniques for the treatment of gingival recession.

References

[1] Wennström J, Pini Prato GP. Mucogingival therapy . In: Lindhe J, Karring T, Lang NP, eds. *Clin. Periodontol. Implant. Dent*, Copenhagen. Munksgaard. 1997:569-591.

[2] American Academy of Periodontology. Proceedings of the World Workshop in Periodontics. *Ann. Periodontol.* 1996 Chicago, The Academy.

[3] Miller PD Jr. Root coverage grafting for regeneration and aesthetics. *Periodontol* 2000. 1993; 1:118–127.

[4] Roccuzzo M, Bunino M, Needleman I and Sanz M. Periodontal plastic surgery for treatment of localized gingival recessions: a systematic review. *J. Clin. Periodontol.* 2002; 29(Suppl. 3): 178–194.

[5] Karring T, Lang NP, Löe H. The role of gingival connective tissue in determining epithelial differentiation. *J. Periodont Res.* 1975; 10:1-11.

[6] Edel A. Clinical evaluation of free connective tissue grafts used to increase the width of keratinized gingiva. *J. Clin. Periodontol* 1974; 1:185-196.

[7] Langer B, Langer L. Sub epithelial connective tissue graft technique for root coverage. *J. Periodontol.* 1985; 56:715-720.

[8] Yukna RA, Tow HD, Carroll PB. Evaluation of the use of freeze-dried skin allografts in the treatment of human mucogingival problems. *J. Periodontol.* 1977; 48:187-193.

[9] Silverstein LH, Callan DP. An Acellular Dermal Matrix allograft substitute for palatal donor tissue. *Post Grad. Dent.* 1996; 3; 14-21.

[10] Shulman J. Clinical evaluation of an Acellular Dermal allograft for increasing the zone of attached gingiva. *Pract. Periodontics Aesthet Dent.* 1997; 8(2)201-208.

[11] Bastista EL Jr, Batista FC, Novaes AB Jr. Managing soft tissue fenestrations in bone grafting surgery with an Acellular Dermal Matrix. A casereport. *Int. J. Oral Max Implants* 2001; 16[6]:875-879.

[12] Harris RJ. Root coverage with a connective tissue with partial thickness double pedicle graft and an Acellular Dermal Matrix graft. A clinical and histological evaluation of a case report. *J. Periodontol.* 1998; 69:1305-1311.

[13] Dodge JR, Henderson R, Greenwell H. Root coverage without a palatal donor site using an acellular dermal graft. Periodont Insights 1998:5:5-9.

[14] Tal H. Subgingival acellular dermal matrix allograft for the treatment of gingival recession. A case report. *J. Periodontol.* 1999; 70:1118; 1124.

[15] Aichelmann Reidy ME, Yukna RA, Evans GH, Nasr HF, Mayer ET. Clinical evaluation of Acellular Allograft dermis for the treatment of human gingival recession. *J. Periodontol.* 2001; 72(8); 998-1005.

[16] Silness J, Loe H. Periodontal disease in pregnancy(II). Corelation between oral hygiene and periodontal conditions. Acta Odontol Scand 1964;22:121-35.

[17] Loe H,Silness J. Periodontal disease in pregnancy(I) Prevalence and severity. *Acta Odontol. Scand* 1963;21: 533-51

[18] Shieh T, Wang H, Neal R, Glickman G, Macneil L. Development and clinical evaluation if a root coverage procedure using a collagen barrier membrane. *J. Periodontol.* 1997; 68:770-778.

[19] Zucchelli G, De Sanctis MD. Treatment of multiple recession-type defects in patients with esthetic demands. J Periodontol 2000; 71:1506-1514.

[20] Arweiler N, Auschill T, Donos N, Sculean A. Antibacterial effect of an enamel matrix protein derivative on in vivo dental biofilm vitality. *Clin. Oral. Invest* (2002) 6:205–209.

[21] Paolantonio M, Dolci M, Esposito P, D' Archivio D, Lisanti L. Subpedicle Acellular dermal matrix graft and autogenous connective tissue graft in the treatment of gingival recessions. A comparative 1-year clinical study. *J. Periodontol.* 2002 Nov; 73(11): 1299-1307.

[22] Novaes AB Jr, Grisi DC, Molina GO, Souza SLS, Taba M Jr, Grisi MFM. Comparative 6 month clinical study of sub epithelial connective tissue graft and acellular dermal matrix graft for treatment of gingival recession. *J. Periodontol* 2001; 72:1477-1484.

[23] Harris RJ. A comparative study of root coverage obtained with an Acellular Dermal matrix versus a connective tissue graft: Results of 107 Recession Defects in 50 Consecutively Treated Patients. *Int. J. Perio Rest Dent* 2000; 20:51-59.

[24] Edel A. Clinical evaluation of free connective tissue grafts used to increase the width of keratinized gingiva. *J. Clin. Periodontol.* 1974; 1:185–196.

[25] Cueva MA, Boltchi FE, Hallmon WW, Nunn ME, Rivera-Hidalgo F, Rees T. A Comparative study of coronally advanced flaps with and without the addition of enamel matrix derivative in the treatment of marginal tissue recession. *J. Periodontol.* 2004; 75:949-956.

[26] Shin SH, Cueva MA, Kerns DG, Hallmon WW, Rivera-Hidalgo F, Nunn ME. A comparative study of root coverage using acellular dermal matrix with and without enamel matrix derivative. *J. Periodontol.* 2007; 78:411-421.

[27] Tal H, Moses O, Zohar R, Meir H, Nemcovsky C. Root coverage of advanced gingival recession: A comparative study between acellular dermal matrix allograft and sub epithelial connective tissue grafts. *J. Periodontol.* 2002;73(12):1405-1411.

[28] 28. Rahmani ME Lades MA. Comparative Clinical Evaluation of Acellular Dermal Matrix Allograft and Connective Tissue Graft for the Treatment of Gingival Recession. *J. Contemp. Dent Practice*, 2006 Vol 7(2):1-12.

[29] Borghetti, Gardella JP. Thick Gingival auto graft for the coverage of gingival recession. A Clinical evaluation. *Int. J. Periodontics Rest. Dent.* 1990; 10:216-229.

[30] Wei PC, Laurell L, Geivelis M, Lingen MW, Maddalozzo D. Acellular Dermal Matrix Allografts to achieve increased attached gingiva: Part 1. A clinical study. *J. Periodontol.* 2000; 71(8); 1297-1305.

[31] Bouchard P, Etienne D, Ouhayoun JP. Sub epithelial connective tissue graft in the treatment of gingival recession. A comparative study of 2 procedures. *J. Periodontol* 1994; 65: 929-936.

[32] Harris RJ. Acellular Dermal Matrix used for root coverage. A 18-month follow up observation. *Int. J. Perio Rest Dent* 2002; Apr; 22(2); 156-163.

[33] Raetzke PB. Covering localized areas of root exposure employing the “Envelope” technique. *J. Periodontol.* 1985; 56; 397- 402.

[34] Piniprato G, Pagliaro U, Baldi C, Wieri M, Saletta D, Cairo F, Cortellini P. Coronally Advanced flap procedure for root coverage. Flap with tension versus flap without tension: A randomized controlled clinical study. *J. Periodontol* 2000; 71:188-201

[35] Henderson RD, Drisko CH, Greenwell H. Predictable multiple site root coverage using an Acellular Dermal Matrix allograft. *J. Periodontol.* 2001; 72:571-582.

[36] Hwang D, Wang H. Flap Thickness as a Predictor of Root Coverage: A Systematic Review. *J. Periodontol.* 2006, Vol. 77, No. 10, Pages 1625-1634.

[37] Chambrone L, Chambrone D, Pustiglioni FE, Chambrone LA, Lima LA. Can subepithelial connective tissue grafts be considered the gold standard procedure in the treatment of Miller Class I and II recession-type defects? *J. Dent.* 2008 Sep; 36(9): 659-71.

In: A Window on Surgery and Orthodontics
Editor: Giuseppe Alessandro Scardina

ISBN: 978-1-62808-948-6

Chapter V

Understanding and Evaluating the Role of Local Anaesthesia in Dentistry: A Brief Review

Preetinder Singh*
Periodontology and Oral Implantology,
Department of Periodontology and Oral Implantology,
Swami Devi Dyal Hospital and Dental College,
Barwala, Distt. Panchkula (Haryana) India

Abstract

Local anesthesia forms the major part of pain-control techniques in dentistry. The prevention and elimination of pain during dental treatment has benefited patients, their doctors, and dental hygienists, enabling the dental profession to make tremendous therapeutic advances that would otherwise have been impossible. Introduced in the late 1940s, the amide local anesthetics represent the most used drugs in dentistry. Local anesthetics also represent the safest and most effective drugs in all of medicine for the prevention and management of pain. They are also accompanied by various adverse effects which should be well known and be able to controlled by the clinician. The article reviews the types of agents uses as local anesthetics and their effects on the human body.

Clinical Significance: Beneficial to all the dental students as well as practitioners in clinical field of dentistry as the local anesthetic agents form an inseparable part of daily dental practice.

Keywords: Anesthesia, dental; anesthetics, local/adverse effects; pharmacology; vasoconstrictor agents

* Corresponding Postal Address: Dr.Preetinder Singh, H.no 28, Sangam Enclave, Sector 48-A, Chandigarh (160047) INDIA. Contact no. : 0091-9915652946. Email : preetinder.perio@yahoo.com.

Local anesthetics are the most commonly used drugs in dentistry. Pain and dentistry are often synonymous in the minds of patients, especially those with poor dentition due to multiple extractions, periodontal disease requiring surgery, or symptomatic teeth requiring endodontic therapy. Dental practitioners identify a good anesthetic as one that allows them to focus solely on operative procedures without distractions from pain-induced patient movements. The everyday practice of dentistry is therefore based upon achieving adequate local anesthesia. Research has shown that the fear of pain associated with dentistry is closely associated with the most common method for blocking pain during dental procedures-intraoral administration of local anesthetics. This is considered aversive due to the pain associated with the injection and the perceived threat of needle puncture prior to the injection [1]. Another survey finding was that those individuals who reported themselves as highly fearful of dentistry were worried about receiving oral injections and demonstrated an association between high dental anxieties and missed or delayed appointments [2].

This article provides a brief overview of local anesthetics to reinforce clinician's knowledge of these agents.

History of Local Anesthesia

The history of local anesthesia started in 1859, when cocaine was isolated by Niemann. In 1884, the opthalmologist Koller was the first, who used cocaine for topical anesthesia in ophthalmological surgery. In 1884, regional anesthesia in the oral cavity was first performed by the surgeon Halsted, when he removed a wisdom tooth without pain. However, a number of adverse effects were observed with the clinical use of cocaine. Thus, other local anesthetic agents had to be developed. In 1905, Einhorn reported the synthesis of procaine, which was the first ester-type local anesthetic agent. Procaine was the most commonly used local anesthetic for more than four decades. In 1943, Löfgren synthesized lidocaine, which was the first modern local anesthetic agent, since it is an amide-derivate of diethylamino acetic acid. Lidocaine was marketed in 1948 and is up to now the most commonly used local anesthetic in dentistry worldwide, though other amide local anesthetics were introduced into clinical use: mepivacaine 1957, prilocaine 1960, bupivacaine 1963. In 1969, articaine was synthesized by the chemist Muschaweck and was approved in 1975 as a local anesthetic in Germany.

The use of reversible local anesthetic chemical agents is the most common method to achieve pain control in dental practice [3]. Some ideal properties of local anesthetics are as follows:

- Specific action
- Reversible action
- Rapid onset of action
- Suitable duration of action
- Active whether applied topically or injected
- Nonirritant
- Causes no permanent damage
- No systemic toxicity
- High therapeutic ratio

- Chemically stable and a long shelf life
- Ability to combine with other agents without loss of properties
- Sterilizable without loss of properties
- Nonallergenic
- Nonaddictive

Pharmacology

Local anesthesia is induced when propagation of action potentials is prevented, such that sensation cannot be transmitted from the source of stimulation, such as a tooth or the periodontium, to the brain. Local anesthetics work by blocking the entry of sodium ions into their channels, thereby preventing the transient increase in permeability of the nerve membrane to sodium that is required for an action potential to occur. Structurally, local anesthetics have specific fundamental features in common. These include a lipophilic group, joined by an amide or ester linkage to a carbon chain which, in turn, is joined to a hydrophilic group. Local anesthetics are classified by these amide or ester linkages.

Different drugs have different proportions of hydrophilic and lipophilic components. These differences modify the characteristics and/or the properties of the anesthetic agents in the following ways:

- Intrinsic anesthetic potency: the minimum concentration of local anesthetic required to reduce the nerve amplitude by half its amplitude within 5 minutes. It is a measure of pharmacologic action of the agent.
- Onset of anesthesia: the onset of anesthesia is dependent on the speed at which the agent passes through the tissue, the proximity of site of injection to the nerve to be anesthetized, and the diameter of the nerve fibers. Thin fibers are anesthetized more rapidly as compared with thick fibers, possibly because the nodes of Ranvier are closer together.
- Duration of action: duration of action of anesthesia is dependent on the rate of diffusion along a concentration gradient away from its site of action-the ion channels in the nerves.
- Effects on other tissues including toxicity: the functions of lipid-containing organs and tissues such as the brain and heart may be affected by high levels of local anesthetics.
- Rate of degradation, both systemically and locally: most amide local anesthetic agents are broken down by hepatic dealkylation and hydrolysis and are subsequentially conjugated with glucuronic acid and excreted in the urine. Esters are metabolized by esterases that are widely distributed in the body.

The most important factors affecting onset are pH of the tissue and pKa of the drug. The pH may drop in sites of infection, which causes onset to be delayed or even prevented. Clinically, there are no significant differences in pKa among the amides, with the exception of bupivacaine, which has a slightly higher pKa and hence a slower onset of action.

Proximity of the deposition of local anesthetic to the nerve can also be a factor, which is why infiltration is associated with rapid onset whereas the Gow-Gates block is relatively slow. Nerve morphology is a factor, in that the relatively thin pain fibres are usually anesthetized readily. Within limits, higher concentration and greater lipid solubility improve onset to a small degree.

Blood Levels

The blood level of local anesthetic agent following injection is a function of both rate of absorption from the site of injection and uptake into the systemic circulation, and its removal through distribution from the vascular compartment into tissue compartments, and elimination via metabolic and excretory pathways. If toxic levels are reached or exceeded, local anesthetics may cause toxic signs and symptoms, which are mainly referable to the Central Nerve System (CNS) and to the Cardiac Vascular System (CVS).

Pharmacokinetic parameters, including maximum serum levels, time of maximum serum levels and elimination half time, are important to estimate the risk of systemic intoxication following injection and to recommend maximal dose in single and repeated injection. The absorption and subsequent blood level of local anesthetic agents are related to the total dose of drug administered. For most agents, there is a linear relationship between the amount of drug administered and the resultant peak of anesthetic blood level.

The peak of anesthetic blood level does not appear to be related to either the concentration or volume of the local anesthetic solution employed. The vasocontrictor (e. g., 1:200,000 epinephrine) significantly reduces the peak of blood levels of lidocaine and mepivacaine, while the peak levels of bupivacaine and prilocaine appear not to be influenced by the addition of a vasoconstrictor substance. After a single injection of a local anesthetic solution, serum levels of the local anesthetic increase fast. After attaining a peak concentration, the serum levels decrease depending on the distribution, metabolization and elimination. The rate of disappearance from blood usually is described in terms of the time required for a 50 % reduction in blood concentration. Peak serum levels, time of peak levels and elimination half-time are different in various local anesthetics and depend on physicochemical characteristics and the way of metabolization.

Failure of Anesthesia

Failure of local anesthetics to achieve profound analgesia may be related to:

- inaccurate anatomic placement of local anesthetic solution
- placing too little solution
- allowing insufficient time for it to diffuse and take effect
- injecting into inflamed or infected tissues
- using an outdated or improperly stored anesthetic solution.

It is recommended that a local anesthetic not be injected in infected tissue because of the risk of spreading the infection and the increased probability of achieving less than effective anesthetic results owing to the low pH within the infected tissue maintaining the ionized, non lipid- soluble state to the anesthetic.

Adverse Reactions

Complications of local anesthetic administration include both local effects and systemic effects [4].

Allergic Reactions and Toxicity

Patient reports of allergic reactions to local anesthetics are fairly common, but investigation shows that most of these are of psychogenic origin. [5, 6] True allergy to an amide is exceedingly rare, whereas the ester procaine is somewhat more allergenic. A patient may be allergic to other compounds in the anesthetic cartridge. For example, methylparabens are preservatives necessary for multidose vials and were present in dental cartridges in the past. They are no longer included as dental cartridges are single-use items. Allergy to para-aminobenzoic acid would rule out use of esters and methylparabens. It may be best to avoid a vasoconstrictor if there is a true documented allergy to sulfites, as metabisulfite is added as an antioxidant whenever vasoconstrictor is present. Toxic complications as a result of an overdose of local anaesthetic solution, resulting in dangerously high concentrations in the brain, are usually produced only by rapid injection directly into a blood vessel [7]. It should be remembered that for fit adults the recommended maximum safe dose of 2% lignocaine in 1:80 000 adrenaline is fourand- a-half 2 or 2. 2 ml cartridges (180 to 198 mg lignocaine); for 3% prilocaine, and felypressin 0. 03 i. u. /ml, the maximum safe dose is 400 mg (six 2 ml cartridges). [8] Some studies have shown that intravascular injection may occur in between 3 and 12% of cases [9]. To avoid accidents with potentially hazardous results, routine aspiration is essential. As the anaesthetic solutions of the amide type (e. g. lignocaine and prilocaine) rely on the liver for hydrolysis and metabolism before elimination, any patient with seriously impaired liver function is in danger of inadequate elimination of the solution: a normal volume of anaesthetic will become potentially toxic in such people. The final route for elimination of the metabolized anaesthetic solution is excretion in the urine and so any patient with impaired renal function will also be unable to eliminate these products and be predisposed to toxic accumulation. The effects of the build up of the local anaesthetic or its breakdown products may occur in two distinct phases: an initial central nervous system stimulation followed by a marked cerebral depression. Stimulation is noted by symptoms ranging from increased anxiety, restlessness, hallucinations to increased depth and rate of respiration, gagging, vomiting and even the risk of severe cortical stimulation resulting in tremors and convulsions. However, with the onset of medullary depression these symptoms will fade as there will be a lapse into unconsciousness, a drop in the blood pressure and a marked reduction in the respiratory rate. Death would result from respiratory failure.

Psychogenic Reactions

Anxiety-induced events are by far the most common adverse reaction associated with local anesthetics in dentistry. These may manifest in numerous ways, the most common of which is syncope. In addition, they may present with a wide variety of symptoms, including hyperventilation, nausea, vomiting and alterations in heart rate or blood pressure. Psychogenic reactions are often misdiagnosed as allergic reactions and may also mimic them, with signs such as urticaria, edema and bronchospasm.

Methemoglobinemia

This uncommon adverse reaction is associated most notably with prilocaine but may also occur with articaine or the topical anesthetic benzocaine. Methemoglobinemia is induced by an excess of the metabolites of these drugs and manifests as a cyanotic appearance that does not respond to the administration of 100% oxygen. Cyanosis becomes apparent when methemoglobin levels are low, but symptoms of nausea, sedation, seizures and even coma may result when levels are very high. [10] Prilocaine, articaine and benzocaine are best avoided in patients with congenital methemoglobinemia.

Facial Nerve Palsy

The most common neurological complication following an inferior alveolar nerve block is a facial nerve palsy [11-16] Patients with a peripheral facial nerve palsy exhibit the following signs:

- generalized weakness of the ipsilateral side of the face;
- inability to close the eyelids;
- obliteration of the nasolabial fold;
- drooping of the corner of the mouth; and
- deviation of the mouth to the unaffected side

Facial nerve palsy following inferior alveolar nerve block may appear immediately or be delayed. The immediate (transient) palsy generally recovers within 3 hours of administration of the local anaesthetic. It is probably due to anaesthesia of the facial nerve trunk as a result of an abnormal nerve anatomy such as passage of the nerve along the deep surface of the parotid gland. Alternatively, it may be caused by a congenital abnormality such as the gland failing to envelop the nerve and its divisions, thus increasing its chances of direct exposure to local anaesthetic solution. Delayed-onset facial palsy occurs after several hours (and in some cases many days) after the administration of the anaesthetic. Some hypotheses have been put forward to explain this.

1. The anaesthetic solution or its breakdown products stimulate the sympathetic plexus associated with the external carotid artery. From the external carotid artery, fibres of

this plexus continue in association with the stylomastoid artery as it passes into the parotid gland. The stimulation of the stylomastoid sympathetic plexus causes a delayed reflex spasm of the vasa nervorum of the facial nerve, leading to ischaemic neuritis and secondary oedema. The origin of these sympathetic fibres is in the superior cervical ganglion which gives rise to lateral, medial and anterior branches. Of these, it is the anterior branches that pass onto the common and external carotid arteries to form plexuses that accompany the blood vessels. [11]

2. The mechanical action of the needle itself may lead to stimulation of the sympathetic plexus associated with the external carotid artery [13].

Paresthesia

Prolonged anesthesia or paresthesia of the tongue or lip are known risks of surgical procedures such as extractions but may also occur following nonsurgical dentistry. Most of these reactions are transient and resolve within 8 weeks, but they may become permanent. Articaine and prilocaine were reported as more likely than other anesthetics to be associated with paresthesia, a difference that was statistically significant when their distribution of use was taken into account [17]. Other causes of persistent paraesthesia include direct nerve damage following injection of local anaesthetics contaminated with sterilizing agents or the development of haemorrhage or haematoma around the nerve sheath leading to necrosis of the neural tissue. Direct inferior nerve trauma feels like an electric shock, sometimes causing the patient to suddenly jerk their head. The practitioner should cease the injection immediately if this occurs [18].

Hematoma

The damage of a blood vessel by the tip of a needle may lead to bleeding into the tissues, resulting in the formation of a hematoma. Significant bleeding may produce swelling, act as an irritant to the tissues, and cause pain and trismus. Theoretically, the localized collection of blood becomes an ideal culture medium for bacteria, although infection of a hematoma is unusual.

Total Body Hemiparesis

Inadvertent intravascular injection of local anaesthetic with subsequent retrograde internal movement in branches of the internal carotid artery has been suggested as a mechanism for a reported case of total body hemiparesis 15 minutes following inferior dental nerve block. This comprised ptosis, occipital and neck stiffness, anaesthesia of the right side of the face with dysphasia, and led to complete aphasia and a right hemiparesis. The effects lasted for approximately 45 minutes and were attributed to excess pressure created during the administration of the injection leading to a retrograde flow into the internal carotid artery [19].

Malignant Hyperthermia

Malignant hyperthermia can occur when patients with genetic susceptibility to this condition are exposed to inhalational general anesthetics or succinylcholine, but not to local anesthetics. Previous recommendations, now known to be wrong, precluded the use of specific local anesthetics in these patients. Today it is well accepted that all local anesthetics are safe for patients who are susceptible to malignant hyperthermia.

Adverse Effects of Epinephrine

Depending on the dose, sympathomimetic amines can evoke a variety of systemic reactions. The major systemic effects of injected sympathicomimetic amines involve the cardiovascular system. Heart rate and contractile force increase under the influence of epinephrine. Arterioles and veins are constricted or dilatated, depending on the total dose of epinephrine and the receptors activated. Cardiovascular responses of epinephrine often include tachycardia, mild hypertension, and occasionally premature ventricular contractions. The majority of adverse reactions are mild and short of duration. Headache can result in the rare occurrence of a severe hypertensive response. Since moderate doses of epinephrine lower total peripheral resistance, the mean arterial pressure may remain unchanged or become slightly reduced. In sensitive patients or under certain conditions, epinephrine may cause pronounced tachycardia or hypertension and may elicit dangerous cardiac arrhythmias, angina pectoris attack or myocardial infarction.

Horner's Syndrome

A rare complication following an inferior dental nerve block, reported by Campbell et al. [20] is the development of Horner's syndrome. This arose due to penetration of the local anaesthetic through the lateral pharyngeal and prevertebral spaces, causing blockade of the stellate ganglion.

The features of the syndrome include:

- flushing of the face on the same side;
- ptosis of the eyelid;
- vasodilatation of the conjunctiva; pupillary constriction; and
- (occasionally) a rash over the neck, face, shoulder and arm of the ipsilateral side.

Paralysis of Ombinations of Cranial Nerves

Use of techniques such as Gow-Gates may result in local anaesthetic, which is deposited in a superior position, gaining access to the cavernous sinus following inadvertent intravenous injection. Consequently, reports have been made of transient paralysis of combined cranial nerves III, IV and VI, leading to immobility of the ipsilateral eyeball, diplopia, ptosis of the eyelid and—in contrast to Horner's syndrome—a dilated pupil.

Careful aspiration and direction of the needle to an area with fewer large-bore blood vessels such as the lateral aspect of the condyle are recommended to avoid this complication. [21]

Temporary Blindness

Temporary blindness has been reported following posterior alveolar nerve block due to a large quantity of local anaesthetic under great pressure diffusing through the inferior orbital fissure and coming into contact with the optic nerve [22].

Sudden Unilateral Deafness

There has also been a report of sudden unilateral deafness following dental procedures involving inferior dental nerve blocks. The suggested explanation implies that the venous systems within the mandibular region provide access for the anaesthetic to the middle ear and that this, due to the added vasoconstrictor, results in localized vasospasm of the cochlear division of the internal auditory artery, leading to dysfunction of the cochlear nerve. [23]

Cardiovascular Disease Patients

The patients with ischemic heart disease (angina pectoris, previous myocardial infarction) or who have had previous cardiac surgery orcirculatory dysfunction such as cardiac failure, show higher plasma levels of lidocaine when compared with healthy subjects given the same dose. Therefore it is recommended that the maximum safe dose be halved in such patients. [24] Low plasma potassium levels and acidosis also potentiate adverse effects of local anesthetics on the myocardium. [4]

The role of the dental practitioner is to maintain an airway, ensure the patient is breathing and monitor cardiac activity. Whilst performing these primary measures the practitioner should summon help and contact the nearest casualty department. Placing the patient supine and administering oxygen will allow monitoring of vital signs (pulse, respiration and blood pressure). Convulsions, which occur in some cases, may need to be treated with a slow (over 2 minutes) intravenous infusion of 10 mg diazepam. The rectal route is an alternative when intravenous access is difficult.

Regional or Systemic Infection

The spread of infection within the perioral tissues can be potentially spread through planes of the head and neck by passage of a needle through an infected area.

Endocarditis Risk

Injections such as the intraligamentary injection can force bacteria into the systemic circulation and cause bacterial endocarditis.

Local Anesthetics during Pregnancy

The adverse drug reactions during pregnancy may affect either the mother or the fetus. Hypersensitivity, allergy, or toxicity reactions in the mother may compromise her health and limit her ability to support a pregnancy.

Fortunately, doses of local anesthetics in dentistry are usually relatively small and are generally unlikely to cause complications during pregnancy. All local anesthetics cross the placenta to some degree. [25-27] Highest concentrations in the fetal circulation follow injection of prilocaine, and the lowest follow bupivacaine, with lidocaine in between. [28, 29]. Felypressin, which is a derivative of vasopressin and is related to oxytocin, has the potential to cause uterine contractions. Although this is a highly unlikely effect at the low dose of felypressin used in local anesthetics, it is best avoided during pregnancy. Lidocaine with epinephrine is commonly used for pregnant dental patients. Although high-dose vasoconstrictors used to manage significant hypotension may be a concern for pregnant patients, the doses of epinephrine used in local anesthetic formulations for dentistry are so low that they are unlikely to significantly affect uterine blood flow. The benefits of epinephrine or levonordefrin at the concentrations found in dental anesthetic cartridges justify their use.

Local Anesthetics in Children

Available data suggest that adverse reactions in pediatric patients are commonly caused by inadequate dosage reduction. [30] Maximum recommended doses of local anesthetics is based upon the weight of the child, usually expressed as milligrams per kilogram of body weight. For very obese children, the maximum dose should be calculated on the basis of lean body weight or ideal weight, not the true body weight. The specific number of milligrams per kilogram used for calculating the maximum recommended dose differs among the various local anesthetics. Given the concerns regarding toxicity, selection of a low concentration solution appears prudent. Thus, 2% lidocaine with epinephrine 1:100,000 may be the ideal local anesthetic for a child.

Bupivacaine is best avoided in children because of its long duration of soft-tissue anesthesia. There should be no concerns regarding prolonged duration of action due to vasoconstrictor, as it has been shown that soft-tissue anesthesia does not differ significantly between 2% lidocaine with epinephrine 1:100,000 and 3% mepivacaine plain or 4% prilocaine plain [31].

Aging Patients

Aging patients are often suffering from general diseases. Metabolization and elimination of drugs may be reduced and delayed. Thus, cumulation of drugs may be possible if repeated injection is performed. In aging patients, local anesthetics with a fast metabolization should be used.

Conclusion

The selection of a local anesthetic for intraoral injection must include considerations of efficacy, safety, and individual patient and operative needs. Drug selection has to consider both components of the anesthetic solution. The local anesthetic agent must have a high intrinsic activity and a low systemic toxicity. The complications due to the local anaesthetic solution itself demand knowledge of the pharmacology of the drugs used and an awareness that it is important to obtain an accurate medical history. Use of epinephrine can be justified for most dental procedures, but it may be necessary to reduce the dose for patients receiving specific medications and those with cardiovascular disease.

References

[1] Rosenberg ES. A computer-controlled anesthetic delivery system in a periodontal practice: patient satisfaction and acceptance. *J. Esthet Restor. Dent.* 2002;14:39-46.

[2] Robinson PD, Pitt Ford TR, McDonald F. *Local anesthesia in dentistry*. London: Reed Educational and Professional Publishing; 2000.

[3] Haas DA. An update on local anesthetics in dentistry. *J. Can Dent. Assoc*. 2002;68:546-551.

[4] Chen AH. Toxicity and allergy to local anesthesia. *J. Calif Dent Assoc*. 1998;26:683-692.

[5] Gall H, Kaufmann R, Kalveram CM. Adverse reactions to local anesthetics: analysis of 197 cases. *J. Allergy Clin. Immunol.* 1996; 97(4):933-7.

[6] Rood JP. Adverse reaction to dental local anaesthetic injection —'allergy' is not the cause. *Br. Dent J.* 2000; 189(7):380-4.

[7] Aldrete JA, Narang R, Sada T et al. Reverse carotid flow: a possible explanation for some reactions to local anaesthetics. *J. Am. Dent Assoc* 1977; 94: 1142.

[8] Meechan J. How to avoid local anaesthetic toxicity. *Br. Dent J.* 1998; 184: 334-335.

[9] Schiano AM, Strambi RC. Frequency of accidental intravascular injections in dental practice. *Oral Surg* 1964; 17: 178.

[10] Wilburn-Goo D, Lloyd LM. When patients become cyanotic: acquired methemoglobinemia. *J. Am. Dent. Assoc* 1999; 130(6):826-81.

[11] Tiwari IB, Keane T. Hemifacial palsy after inferior dental block for dental treatment. *BMJ* 1970; 1:798.

[12] Gray RLM. Peripheral facial nerve paralysis of dental origin. *Br. J. Oral Surg*. 1978-79; 16: 143-150.

[13] Ling KC. Peripheral facial nerve paralysis after local dental anaesthesia. *Oral Surg. Oral Med. Oral Pathol.* 1985; 60: 23-24.

[14] Miles EG. Facial palsy in the dental surgery. Case report and a review. *Aust. Dent J.* 1992; 37: 262-265.

[15] Bernsen BLJA. Peripheral facial nerve palsy after local upper dental anaesthesia. *Eur. Neurol.* 1993;33: 90-91.

[16] Shaib A, Lee MA. Recurrent peripheral facial nerve palsy after dental procedures. *Oral Surg Oral Med. Oral Pathol* 1990; 70: 738-740.

[17] Haas DA, Lennon D. A 21 year retrospective study of reports of paresthesia following local anesthetic administration. *J. Can Dent Assoc.* 1995; 61(4):319-20, 323-6, 329-30.

[18] Malamed SF. *Handbook of Local Anaesthesia*, 3rd ed. St Louis: Mosby-Year Book, 1990; pp. 160-218,245-257.

[19] Weinberg A et al. Transient hemiparesis following mandibular nerve anaesthesia. *J. Dent Res.* 1984; 63:549.

[20] Campbell RL, Mercuri LG, Van Sickels J. Cervical sympathetic block following intraoral local anaesthesia. *Oral Surg. Oral Med. Oral Pathol.* 1979;47: 223-226.

[21] Fish LR, McIntire DN, Johnson L. Temporary paralysis of cranial nerves III, IV and VI after a Gow-Gates injection. *J. Am. Dent Assoc* 1989; 119:127-130.

[22] Cooley RL and Cottingham AJ Jr. Ocular complications from local anaesthetic injections. *Gen. Dent* 1979; 27: 40.

[23] Farrell RW, Pemberton MN, Parker AJ, Buffin JT. Sudden deafness after dental surgery. *BMJ* 1991;303: 1034.

[24] Preshaw PM, Rowson JE. The use of lignocaine local anesthetic. *Br. Dent J.* 1996;181:240.

[25] Pertl C, Heinemann A, Pertl B, et al. The pregnant patient in dental care. Survey results and therapeutic guidelines. *Schweiz Monatsschr Zahnmed.* 2000; 110:37-46.

[26] Lawrenz DR, Whitley BD, Helfrick JF. Considerations in the management of maxillofacial infections in the pregnant patient. *J. Oral Maxillofac Surg.* 1996;54:474-485.

[27] Avraamides EJ, Craen RA, Gelb AW. Anesthetic management of a pregnant, post liver transplant patient for dental surgery. *Anesth Intens Care.* 1997;25:68-70.

[28] Johnson CG. Local anesthetics and pregnancy. *J. Am \Dent Assoc.* 1985;110:302.

[29] Watson AK. Local anesthetics in pregnancy. *Br . Dent J.* 1989;166:36.

[30] Hunter ML, Hood CA, Hunter B, Kingdon A. Oral health advice: reported experience of mothers of children aged 5 years and under referred for extraction of teeth under general anesthesia. *Int. J. Pediatr Dent.* 1998;8:13-27.

[31] Hersh EV, Hermann DG, Lamp CJ, Johnson PD, MacAfee KA. Assessing the duration of mandibular soft tissue anesthesia. *J. Am. Dent. Assoc* 1995; 126(11):1531-6.

In: A Window on Surgery and Orthodontics
Editor: Giuseppe Alessandro Scardina ISBN: 978-1-62808-948-6

Chapter VI

Supernumerary Teeth: A Review and Case Report

Jogani Vivek**, *P. Poornima and Subba V. Reddy
Department of Pedodontics and Preventive Dentistry,
College of Dental Sciences, Davangere, India

Abstract

Supernumerary tooth (ST) is a developmental anomaly and has been argued to arise from multiple aetiologies. These teeth may remain embedded in the alveolar bone or can erupt into the oral cavity. When it remains embedded, it may cause disturbance to the developing teeth. The erupted ST might cause aesthetic and/or functional problems especially if it is situated in the maxillary anterior region. This case involves an 8-year-old male with inverted tuberculate rudimentary right ST located in midpalate region and a left ST erupted palatal to left maxillary central incisor.

Keywords: Mesiodens, impacted, supernumerary tooth, dental anomaly

Clinical Significance: The case presented herein was considered to be rare, since the child complained of unusual hindrance to his tongue while swallowing. This could be attributed to its position of the impacted supernumerary tooth and bulge into the oral cavity.

Development of the tooth is a continuous process with a number of physiologic growth processes and various morphologic stages interplay to achieve the tooth's final form and structure. Interference with the stage of initiation, a momentary event, may result in single or

* Address for correspondence: Dr. Jogani Vivek C, Post-Graduate student, Department of Pedodontics and Preventive dentistry, College of Dental Sciences, Davangere. E-mail: vivekdecent19@gmail.com. Ph- +919986323103, +919353071995.

multiple missing teeth or supernumerary teeth (ST). [1] Teeth formed in excess of the normal number are termed supernumerary. ST occurs in 0. 3 %-0. 8% in the primary dentition and 1. 5%-3. 5% in the permanent dentition [2]. These may occur singly, in multiple, unilaterally or bilaterally, and in maxilla, the mandible or both.

Maxillary midline supernumeraries (mesiodens) are the most common type, followed by maxillary lateral incisors, and mandibular third premolars [3]. While there is no significant sex distribution in primary ST, males are affected approximately twice as frequently as females in the permanent dentition [4].

ST can be classified according to their location in the dental arch: mesiodens, paramolar and distomolar or according to their morphological forms: conical, tuberculate, supplemental and odontome [5]. If a supernumerary primary tooth is present clinically, a supernumerary permanent tooth is often evident radiographically [6] Primosh (1981) classified supernumerary into two types according to their shape as supplemental (eumorphic) and rudimentary (dysmorphic). [7] The ST position can be recorded as 'between central incisors' and 'overlap' and its orientation can be described as 'vertical', 'inverted' and 'transverse'[8].

The aetiology of the ST however remains unclear [7]. The phylogenetic reversion (atavism) theory, postulated that mesiodens represented a phylogenetic relic of extinct ancestors who had 3 central incisors. This theory has been largely discarded by embryologists. The dichotomy theory suggests that the tooth bud is split to create 2 teeth, one of which is the mesiodens. Supporters of this theory believe that dichotomy represents complete gemination, which also occurs frequently in the anterior maxilla. According to the most accepted hyperactivity of dental lamina theory, remnants of the dental lamina or palatal offshoots of active dental lamina are induced to develop into an extra tooth bud, which results in a ST.

Genetic and environmental factors have been proposed for ST. Brook (1984) in his study among 1115 children aged 11-14-years-old showed that ST are more common in the relatives of affected children than the general population [9] Autosomal dominant inheritance with incomplete penetration has been the proposed genetic theory [10] A sex-linked pattern has also been proposed, as males are affected twice as frequently as females [1]. The presence of ST may be part of developmental disorders such as Cleft lip and palate, cleidocranial dysostosis, Gardner's syndrome, Ehlers Danlos syndrome, Incontinentia Pigmenti and Tricho-Rhino-Phalangeal syndrome [11].

Most problems associated with mesiodens are related to altered growth and development in the area. Common sequelae include over-retention of primary teeth, impaction or delayed eruption of permanent teeth, dilacerations or abnormal root development, and/or abnormal crowding or spacing of the anterior teeth. The less frequent problems are root resorption of adjacent teeth, dentigerous cyst formation, and nasal eruption of inverted ST [7]

Treatment of mesiodens centres on several factors and consideration of these variables will determine whether to treat the supernumerary early or to observe the condition [12]. The first factor is the child's age. In the very young child the ability to tolerate a surgical procedure is of major concern. The benefit of early treatment must be weighed against the long-term effect that any unpleasant experience may have.

Second is the stage of dental development of the surrounding definition and proximity of the mesiodens to the permanent incisors. In cases of immature root development, consideration must be given to the risk of surgical trauma to the developing roots of the permanent incisors and the potential of altering future dental development. Mesiodens that are intimately positioned with the developing permanent incisors may either alter the permanent bud positionally, impede eruption, and/or alter root development; whereas, removal of this same ST may cause the same sequelae through surgical trauma. In instances where the surgical approach jeopardizes the viability of sensitive developing tissue, it may be appropriate to delay treatment.

Lastly, one must evaluate the relative position of the mesiodens within the premaxilla. Assessment of access to the supernumerary must be considered in relation to the amount of bone removal and potential damage to existing incisors. In children, eruption of mesiodens is possible and, although complete eruption is infrequent, some mesiodens may erupt partially so that a more favourable surgical approach may be attained with time.

Case Report

An 8-year-old boy was referred to the Department of Paediatric Dentistry with a chief complain of unusual discomfort while swallowing and presence of an extra front tooth. There was no history of tumour or trauma in this patient. Being born to non-consanguineous parents, the patient's health status was excellent.

Oral findings: The intraoral examination confirmed the patient's chief complaint. It revealed one erupted eumorphic ST palatal to upper left central incisor. Clinical examination revealed a firm swelling fixed to the midpalate of the maxilla in the first permanent molar and second primary molar region (Figure 1). Maxillary anterior spacing was slightly excessive with a 2-3mm midline diastema present and anterior open bite (Figure 2). Carious lesions were evident and treatment was required accordingly.

Investigation: Occlusal radiograph was taken in order to localise the ST and assess the potential surgical approach (Figure 3). Routine laboratory parameters were normal. An upper and lower impression was taken for construction of study model to monitor changes in tooth movement and fabricate a acrylic resin stent to be used post-operatively. Informed parent consent was obtained prior to start of the procedure.

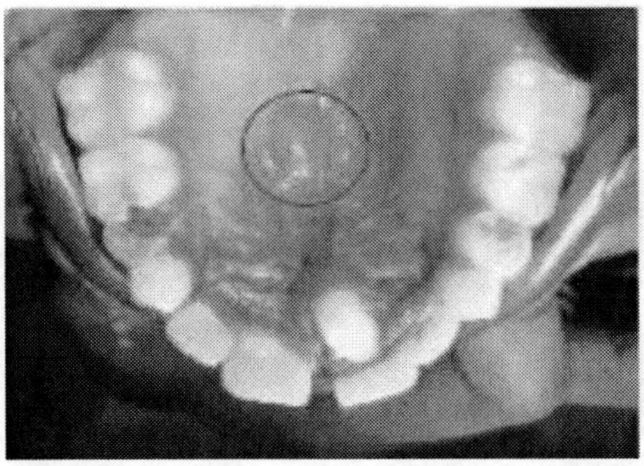

Figure 1. Intra-oral maxillary view showing palatal swelling and erupted left supernumerary tooth.

Treatment: Initially the patient was mildly apprehensive and hence it was decided to extract only the palatally erupted left central incisor. He was given permission to stop treatment by raising his hand if any discomfort was experienced. After local anaesthesia was accomplished the patient seemed much more relaxed. The patient was kept under observation and other routine procedures were carried out until next surgical appointment. After 3 weeks the surgical procedure was performed in the outpatient dental clinic for extraction of the inverted impacted mesiodense. At this visit the patient was cooperative and familiar with the dental environment.

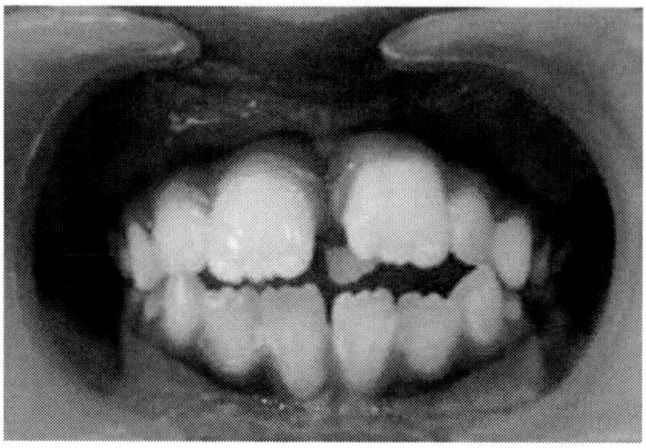

Figure 2. Pre-operative frontal view showing erupted left mesiodense and associated anterior open-bite.

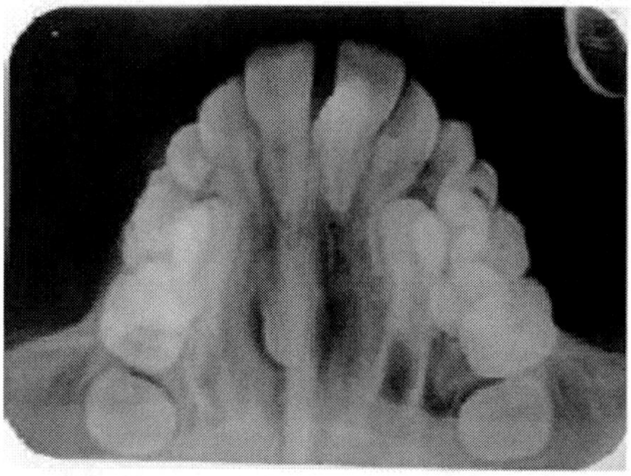

Figure 3. Maxillary true occlusal radiograph showing right inverted supernumerary tooth and left erupted tooth.

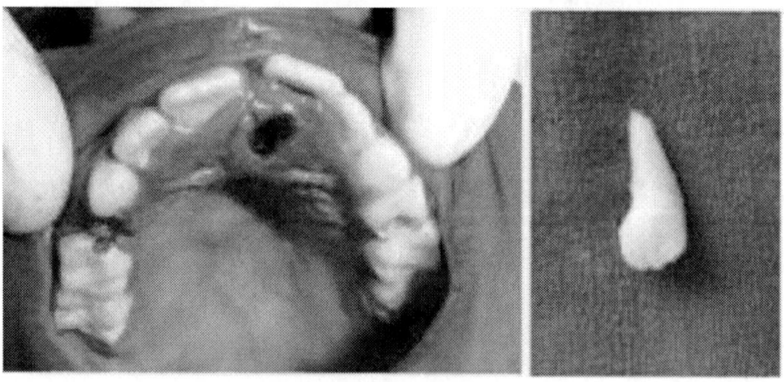

Figure 4. After extraction of erupted left supernumerary tooth.

Local anaesthetic, 2% lidocaine with 1/100,000 epinephrine, was administered slowly via bilateral greater palatine and nasopalatine nerve block with a 27-gauge needle. Using a #15 blade a crevicular incision was made from the distal aspect of maxillary right first permanent molar to the mesial aspect of maxillary left first permanent molar. A full thickness flap then was reflected with a periosteal elevator. The crown was visible clearly. A sterile #8 round bur was used with slow speed to remove the bone which allowed the root to be seen.

With liberal saline irrigation a circular window was made surrounding the tooth. Care was taken to avoid excessive bone removal. At this point it was determined that the mesiodens was in a more horizontal position with the root apex anteriorly positioned and the crown positioned posteriorly. The tooth was then luxated with an elevator. Although mobile, the larger contour of the crown impeded final removal. Following additional circumferential expansion of the bony window, delivery of the ST with dilacerated root was accomplished. The mesiodens measured 13 mm in length (figure 5a).

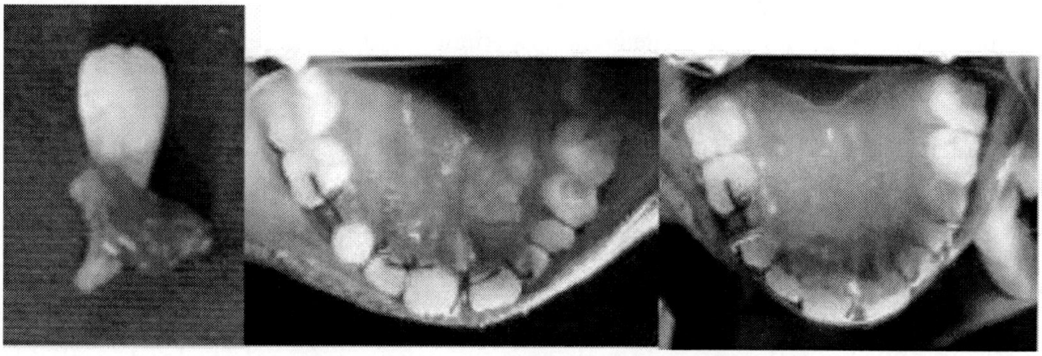

Figure 5. Extracted ST with dilacerated root and Post-operative view after suture placement and stent in place.

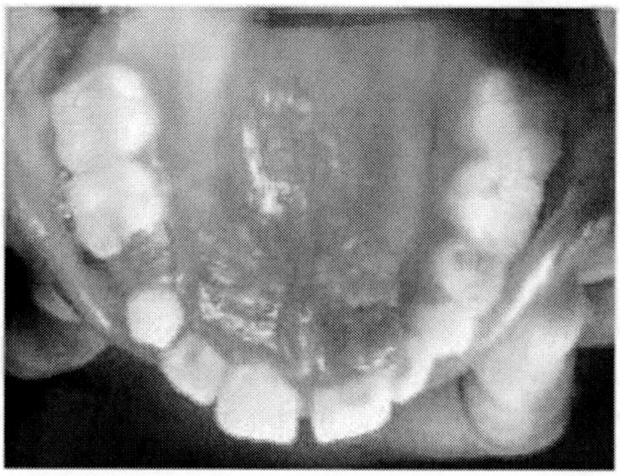

Figure 6. Post-operative view after uneventful healing.

The extraction site was gently curetted, irrigated with saline, and the wound closed with 8 interrupted interdental 4-0 silk sutures (figure 5b). The patient tolerated the procedure comfortably. Postoperative pain was controlled with a paediatric dose ibuprofen. A prefabricated stent was inserted to allow the flap to stay in position and aid in healing (figure 5c). The patient's recovery was uneventful with no usual signs or symptoms reported.

The sutures were removed 1 week postoperatively with normal healing at the surgical site. (6). Initiation of comprehensive orthodontic treatment, previously discussed with the parent was planned in subsequent visits. At the second-month recall, new bone formation was detected radiographically within the extraction sites.

Discussion

A thorough understanding and definitive diagnosis is essential for planning and management of ST. The mesiodense in this patient had probably originated from the permanent dentition tooth bud since in the primary dentition, ST occurred most often in the lateral incisor regions, as opposed to permanent ST, which prevailed in the central incisor regions [13].

Although ST could erupt normally, they generally remain impacted. It has been found that approximately 25% of permanent ST are erupted and remainders are unerupted [11] Nazif et al. reported that only 6% of the impacted mesiodens are found to be in a labial position. The vast majority (80%) are reported to be positioned palatally with the remaining 14% located between the roots of the permanent central incisors [14] Resorption of the adjacent roots by mesiodens or its cyst is a rare complication [15]. In our patient, resorption of the roots was not observed.

There are different schools of thoughts for removal of ST. Extraction of a supernumerary mesiodens in the primary dentition is usually not recommended because supernumerary primary teeth often erupt into the oral cavity and surgical extraction of unerupted teeth may increase the risk of displacing or damaging the developing permanent incisors [12-13, 16] However, extraction during the early mixed dentition stage allows normal eruptive forces to promote spontaneous eruption of the permanent central incisors after the extraction [16-17] Extraction of mesiodens at a time appropriate for promoting self-eruption in the early mixed dentition may result in better alignment of the teeth and may minimise the need for orthodontic treatment.

Delayed treatment involves extraction of the mesiodens when the unerupted central incisor's apex is almost mature, usually around 10 years of age [12]. The later the extraction of the mesiodens, the greater the chance that the permanent tooth either will not spontaneously erupt or will be malaligned when it does erupt. Unfortunately, by this time the forces that cause normal eruption of the incisors are diminished, and surgical exposure and subsequent orthodontic treatment are more frequently required [17] Also, space loss and midline shift of the central incisors may have already occurred by this age, since the lateral incisors will have erupted and may have drifted mesially into the central space [1] Thus, a significant delay in treatment can create the need for more complex surgical and orthodontic management. Also, a survey of 112 ST showed that the teeth in transverse or inverted positions never erupted [18] and it advisable for the supernumerary to be surgically removed since in many instances, supernumerary are associated with disturbances of tooth eruption, midline Diastema or development of a local malocclusion [19].

The case presented herein was considered to be rare, since the child complained of unusual hindrance to his tongue while swallowing. This could be attributed to its position and bulge into the oral cavity. The clinical significance of the inversion is questionable, since left mesiodentes erupted ectopically; whereas right mesiodentes remained intact. Also, the eruption forces acting in a reverse direction could have resulted in the posterior placement of the impacted tooth. However, the occurrence of the erupted mesiodentes was definitely regarded as a contributory factor to the flared teeth in the anterior maxillary region. Fortunately, the post-surgical phase was uneventful, and did not affect commencement of orthodontic therapy after a relatively short follow-up period.

Conclusion

ST usually present with orthodontic problems in children and young adults. Our report documents an unusual swallowing discomfort with impacted inverted mesiodens. Long term monitoring and follow-up is very important when dealing with paediatric dental patient.

Conflict of Interest and Sources of Funding: Nil.

References

[1] Hattab FN, Yassin OM and Rawashdeh MA. Supernumerary teeth: Report of three cases and review of literature. *ASDC J. Dent Child* 1994; 61(5-6): 382-393.

[2] Mason C, Azam N, Holt RD and Rule DC. A retrospective study of unerupted maxillary incisors associated with supernumerary teeth. *Br. J. Oral Maxillofac Surg.* 2000, 38: 6.

[3] Mckibben, D. R. and Bearly, L. J.: Radiographic determination of the prevalence of selected dental anomalies in children. *J. Dent. Child* 1971, 38: 390-398.

[4] Kinirons, M. J., Unerupted premaxillary supernumerary teeth. *Br. Dent J.* 1982, 153: 110.

[5] Mitchell L (1989). Supernumerary teeth. *Dent Update*, 16: 65-69.

[6] Russell KA, Folwarczna MA. Mesiodense- Diagnosis and management of a Common Supernumerary Tooth. *J. Can Dent. Assoc* 2003, 69(6): 362-6.

[7] Primosch RE. Anterior supernumerary teeth- assessment and surgical intervention in children. *Paed. Dent.* 1981; 3: 204-215.

[8] Gregg TA and Kinirons MJ. The effect of the position and orientation of unerupted premaxillary supernumerary teeth on eruption and displacement of permanent incisors. *Int. J. Paed. Dent.* , 1991; 1: 3-7.

[9] Brook AH. A unifying etiological explanation for anomalies of human tooth number and size. *Archs. Oral Biol.* 1984; 29: 373-378.

[10] Sedano HO, Gorlin RJ. Familial occurrence of mesiodense. *Oral Surg. Oral Med. Oral Pathol.* 1969; 27(3): 360-1.

[11] Rajab LD, Hamdan MAM. Supernumerary teeth: review of the literature and a survey of 152 cases. *Int. J. Paed. Dent.* 2002; 12: 244-254.

[12] Henry RJ, Post CA. A labially positioned mesiodens: case report. *Paediatric Dentistry* 1989; 11(1): 59-63.

[13] Humerfelt D, Hurlen B and Humerfelt S. Hyperdontia in children below four years of age: a radiographic study. *ASDC J. Dent. Child* 1985; 52: 121-124.

[14] Nazif MM, Ruffalo RC, Zullo T. Impacted supernumerary teeth: a survey of 50 cases. *J. Am. Dent. Assoc.* 1983; 106: 201-4.

[15] von Arx T. Anterior maxillary supernumerary teeth- A clinical and radiographic study. *Aus. Dent. J.* 1992; 37: 189-95.

[16] Solares R. The complications of late diagnosis of anterior supernumerary teeth: case report. *ASDC J. Dent. Child* 1990; 57(3): 209-211.

[17] Tay F, Pang A, Yuen S. Unerupted maxillary anterior supernumerary teeth: report of 204 cases. *ASDC J. Dent. Child* 1984; 51(4): 289-94.

[18] Liu JF. Characteristics of premaxillary supernumerary teeth: A survey of 112 cases. *ASDC J. Dent for Child* 1995; 62: 262-265.

[19] Tyrologou S, Koch G and Kurol J. Location, complications and treatment of mesiodentes- a retrospective study in children. *Swed. Dent. J.* 2005; 29: 1-9.

In: A Window on Surgery and Orthodontics
Editor: Giuseppe Alessandro Scardina
ISBN: 978-1-62808-948-6

Chapter VII

The Biological Effects of Static Magnetic Field of Commercial Samarium-Cobalt (SmCo5) Orthodontic Magnets on Cultured Escherichia Coli and Staphylococci Aurous

***Hussam M. Abdel-Kader**[*1], **Mohamed I. Aref**[2] **and Sedky W. Yousef**[3]*

[1]Orthodontics, Faculty of Dental Medicine
AlAzhar University and Misr International University (MIU), Cairo, Egypt
[2]Clinical Pathology, Faculty of Medicine, AlAzhar University, Cairo, Egypt
[3]Orthodontic Department, Faculty of Oral and Dental Medicine
Misr International University (MIU), Cairo, Egypt

Abstract

Objective: The current study aimed to investigate the biological effects of the static magnetic fields of commercially available orthodontic samarium-cobalt (SmCo5) magnets on cultured two types of bacteria (E-coli and Staphylococci aurous)

Materials and methods: The study was conducted on: 1. Orthodontic magnets arranged in couples; some of them were fixed in attraction mode and others were fixed in repelling mode with a distance of a 1. 5mm between pole of each two magnets. 2. Three sterilized glass laboratory dishes were plated with Escherichia coli (E. coli) bacteria and another three dishes were plated with Staphylococci aurous. One dish in each group was used as a control group, while the other two dish were used as a test group. On the lid of each test dish, a couple of orthodontic magnets were fixed, one in the attraction mode and the second in repelling mode. 3. The biological effects of the static magnetic field under

* Corresponding author: Prof. Hussam M. Abdel-Kader, Professor of Orthodontics. Mena Garden City 12582, Louvre, Town-house B25. 6 October City. 6 October. Cairo, Egypt. E-mail: hmkader@hotmail.com. Cell phone: +2010-1189-148.

the two conditions, repelling and attraction modes were evaluated after 48 hours. 4. The above motioned steps were repeated for 9 times.

Results: 1. The static magnetic field affected significantly the cell populations in different ways according to the type of cultured cells. 2. The biological effects of the static magnetic field in attraction mode were significantly greater than that recorded in magnets' repelling mode.

Conclusion: 1. Exposure to the static magnetic field of orthodontic magnets for only 48 hours could dramatically affect the growth of Staphylococcus aurous and E-Coli bacteria. 2. The adverse effects of the static magnetic field were significantly higher in attraction mode than that with magnets in repelling mode.

Keywords: Orthodontics, Orthodontic magnets, Static magnetic field, DNA fragmentation

Introduction

Recently, orthodontic magnets have been commercially available for clinical use and directed towards maxillary molar distalization, correction of open bite, canine retraction, fixed retention, arch expansion, functional appliances and orthodontic eruption of unerupted teeth [1-11]. Rare earth magnets made from samarium-cobalt (SmCo5) or neodymium-iron-boron (Nd2Fe14B), are the magnets of clinical choice. Magnets readily corrode in the oral environment if they are not protected [12], and an in-vitro study revealed that unprotected orthodontic magnets, exhibited weight loss of about 31. 15% in 25 days [13]. However, in a clinical study, orthodontic magnets showed significant weight loss of about 3. 07% within six months following the loss of a protective acrylic coat within the first month of clinical use. This was accompanied by a significant release of nickel, chromium and ferrous ions [14] as well as significant apoptotic-DNA fragmentation in the patient's cheek mucosa cells.

The adverse biological effect of SmCo5 magnets in clinical use on the oral mucosa cells is a matter of debate. This could be the end results of the released metal corrosion product from the magnets after peeled-off their resin protecting coats especially nickel, cobalt and samarium and/or the effects of their static magnetic fields. The biological effect of the static magnetic field of the magnets was considered by many investigators [15-20]. The effects could be in the form of changes in cell metabolism, structure and growth. When magnets are used in orthodontics, the oral tissues will be exposed to the static magnetic field during the course of their use. The tissues, which were closest to the magnets, are supposed to be the highest tissue to be exposed to the static magnetic field, than the other intraoral tissues in descending orders.

The point of interest is that orthodontic magnets are used in couple; accordingly is the biological effects of the static magnetic field the same in the repelling mode as in the attracting mode? The question is which one could have the stronger biological effects, the scattered magnetic field of repelling magnets or the combined magnetic field of attracting magnets? In the literature it is concluded that, the static magnetic field exposure value for attractive magnets is somewhat higher compared to that of repelling magnets, but the extent of the static magnetic field is wider in case of repelling magnets compared to attracting magnets [21].

In this very interesting study on the extent and flux density of the static magnetic field of samarium cobalt orthodontic magnets the authors concluded that: 1. The maximum flux density was recorded at the magnets poles. 2. Magnets in attractive mode have a flux density of 2. 2 Kg. 3. Magnets in repelling mode have a flux density of 1. 7 Kg. 4. With increased distance from the magnets the flux density decreased rapidly. Finally they reached a final conclusion that "the static magnetic field exposure of surrounding tissues can be assumed to be low, and the conceivable risk of harmful biological effects must be regarded as small and limited when the tested orthodontic magnets are used clinically".

In view of the above illustrated review of literature, the current study was directed to test the null hypothesis that; the static magnetic field of commercial orthodontic magnets could have adverse biological effects on the living cells.

Materials and Methods

The biological effect of static magnetic field of commercial orthodontic magnets on growth and biochemical reaction of cultured two types of bacteria; Escherichia coli (E. coli) and staphylococci aurous (oral flora bacteria), had been undertaken according to the following standard protocol:

1. As we commonly used orthodontic magnets in couple in different clinical orthodontic purposes, new couples of Samarium-cobalt (SmCo5) orthodontic magnets (Ortho Organizer, Inc. 424-200 Magnetic Force System) were used in the current study. In one couple, the orthodontic magnets were fixed in repelling mode (S-S poles); on the other hand, the second couple the magnets was fixed in attractive mode (S-N poles). The distance between the two magnets' poles in the two conditions (repelling and attraction) was kept at 1. 5mm, as they are used clinically. As we used new orthodontic magnets, in the current study, with completely intact protective layer, there is no fear from the effect of metal ion release on our results.
2. Three sterilized laboratory glass dishes with their cover were prepared and filled with triple sugar iron agar containing E-coli bacteria. One dish was used as a control sample group. On the other hand the other two dishes; one dish was used to test the biological effects of static magnetic field with magnets in attraction mode, and the other dish with magnets in repelling mode. Close to the outer margin on the top surface of the glass cover of the test sample two dishes, couple of orthodontic magnets was fixed; one in attraction mode and the second in repelling mode. The distance between the magnets and the cultured bacteria was in the range of one millimeter.
3. Another three sterilized laboratory glass dishes with their cover were prepared and filled with blood agar cultured media containing Staphylococci aurous bacteria. One dish was used as a control sample group. On the other hand the other two dishes; one dish was used to test the biological effects of static magnetic field with magnets in attraction mode, and the other dish with magnets in repelling mode. Close to the outer margin on the top surface of the glass cover of the test sample two dishes, couple of orthodontic magnets was fixed; one in attraction mode and the second in repelling mode. The distance between the magnets and the cultured bacteria was in the range of one millimeter.

4. Ferric salt in the form of hemoglobin was present in cultured agar (E-coli bacteria) at 3% concentration [22, 23].
5. The six dishes were stored in an incubator at fixed temperature of C37 degrees for 48 hours.
6. The biological effects of magnetic field of orthodontic magnets under the two conditions, attraction and repelling modes, on the cultured bacteria; E-coli and Staphylococci aurous bacteria were investigated after 48 hours.
    1. NB: 1. The above mentioned experiments were repeated 9 times for the two types of bacterial cells under investigation; E-coli and Staphylococci aurous, according to the same designed standard protocol for each experiment.
    2. For about three months several pilot studies had been undertaken till the above mentioned two experimental designs were reached and a standardized protocol for each experiment proved to be valid for the current research design.
    3. During the pilot study it was noticed that magnetic field per-se had no significant effect on the cultured two types of cells under investigation; E-coli and Staphylococci aurous. On the other hand, adding traces amount of ferrous ions to the cells' culture medium enhance the effects of the static magnetic field of orthodontic magnets on the cultured cells. Accordingly Ferric salt in the form of Iron Dextrin Complex 50 mg (10 micrometer had been used) was added as a source of iron to the cultured media [22].

Statistical Analysis

The effect of orthodontic magnets on E-coli and Staphylococci aurous, under the two conditions, attraction and repelling modes, had been statistically analyzed. Paired t test was used to test the level of statistical significant changes in the cultured two types of cells under investigation after 48 hours exposure to the static magnetic field of orthodontic magnets fixed in attraction and repelling modes. Probabilities of less than 5% ($P \leq 0.05$) were considered to be statistically significant.

Results

The pilot studies in the current study revealed that the static magnetic field of commercial orthodontic magnets in common clinical orthodontic uses, per-se, had no adverse biological effects on the cultured two types of cultured cells under investigation; Escherichia coli (E. coli) and Staphylococci aurous. On the other hand adding traces of iron in the form of ferric salt to the culture media enhance the adverse biological effects of orthodontic magnets' galvanic field on the cultured two types of cells but in different patterns according to cell type. When the cultured Staphylococci aurous and E-coli was exposed for 48 hours, the experimental period, to the static magnetic field of orthodontic magnets, this exposure was reflected in the form of inhibition of bacterial growth and affecting the biochemical (enzyme) activity of the two cultured bacteria respectively (Figure 1 A, B, C and D).

The effects of static magnetic field of orthodontic magnets on cultured Staphylococci aurous was notice after 48 hours in the form of inhibition of Staphylococci aurous growth under the two condition; attraction and repelling modes (Figure 1 A and B respectively). It was notice that the area facing the orthodontic magnets nearly free from bacterial growth. The effect of static magnetic field of the orthodontic magnets takes more or less festooned area covering around 1/3 of the surface area of the cultured Staphylococci aurous. The center of this area is exactly under the magnets. On the other hand the effect of static magnetic field on the E-coli was observed in the form of significant inhibition of E-coli biochemical activity under the two condition; attraction and repelling modes (Figure 1 C and D respectively). It was observe that the area facing the orthodontic magnets showed significant change in color which denotes significant changes in the enzymatic activity of the bacteria. This effect was in form of concentric waves of different colors covered around 1/3 of the surface area of the cultured E-coli. The center of the waves is exactly under the magnets.

Figures 1 A and B on the one hand and figures 1 C and D on the other hand, shows clearly the difference in the surface topography, outline and form of extension of the affected areas of the cultured Staphylococcus aurous and E-coli respectively, after 48 hours exposure to the static magnetic field of orthodontic magnets under the attraction and repelling modes. These differences could signify the mode and differences in the effects of static magnetic field on the two types of bacteria under investigation.

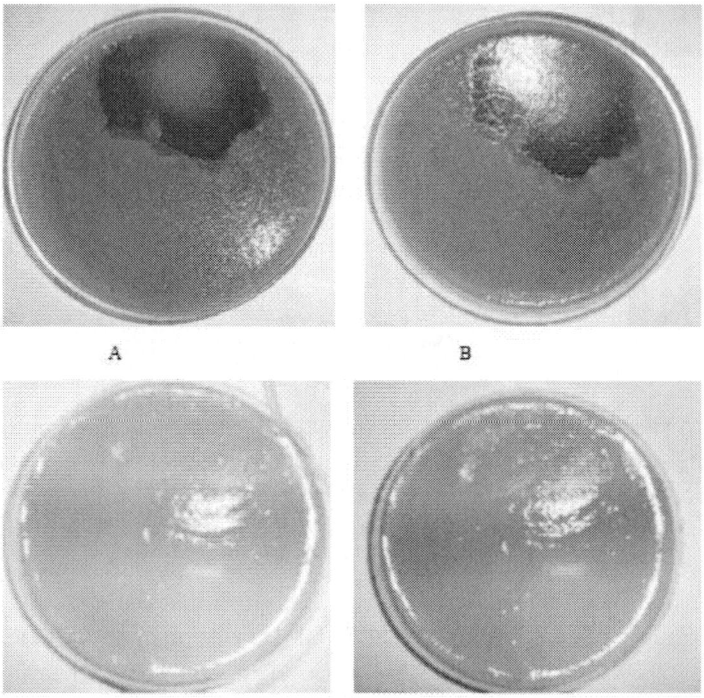

A B

C D

Figure 1. Descriptive statistics the percentage of affected surface area of the cultured two types of bacteria; Staphylococci aurous and E-coli, after exposure to the static magnetic field of orthodontic magnets for 48 hours under the two conditions, repelling and attraction modes, and the level of significance between the two conditions, attraction and repelling modes for the two types of bacteria using paired t test ($P \leq 0.001$).

Figure 1 A and B illustrate the effects of exposing the Staphylococci aurous to the static magnetic field arranged in attraction mode and repelling modes respectively (inhibition of bacterial growth). On the other hand figures C and D illustrate the effects of exposing the E-coli to the static magnetic field arranged in attraction mode and repelling modes respectively (inhibition the enzyme activity of the bacteria). The exposure time for the two types of bacteria to static magnetic field of orthodontic magnets was 48 hours.

The effect of the static magnetic field of orthodontic magnets in repelling mode on inhibiting the E-coli enzymatic activity and Staphylococci aurous growth covered much more extensive area than that in the attraction mode. Regarding the two control sample groups of the Staphylococci aurous and e-coli, no changes could be detected after the 48 hours experimental period.

The percentage of affected surface area of the cultured Staphylococci aurous and E-coli, after exposure to the static magnetic field of orthodontic magnets for 48 hours under the two conditions, repelling and attraction modes were evaluated. It was observe that the percentage of affected surface area of the cultured two types of bacteria in the repelling magnets mode is significantly higher than that recorded in magnets attraction mode where p≤0. 001 (Table 1).

1. Staphylococci aurous			
Repelling (n=9)	Attraction (n=9)	Difference	P value
Mean+/-S. D.	Mean+/- S. D.	Mean diff. +/- S. D diff	
6. 63+/-0. 44	8. 20+/-0. 46	-1. 57+/-0. 88	t = 5. 36 P ≤ 0. 001
2. E-coli			
Repelling (n=9)	Attraction (n=9)	Difference	P value
Mean+/- S. D.	Mean+/- S. D.	Mean diff. +/- S. D diff	
4. 33+/-0. 50	4. 70+/-038	-0. 37+/- 0. 13	t = 8. 31 p ≤ 0. 001

Discussion

In the current study the effect of the static magnetic field of orthodontic magnets, per se, under the repelling-and attraction modes, on living cultured two types of bacterial cells E-coli and Staphylococci aurous bacterial growth and biochemical activity had been investigated.

The effect of static magnetic field of orthodontic magnets on the two types of bacteria under investigation; first on Escherichia coli (E. coli) bacteria was in the form of significant inhibition of bacterial biochemical activity. It was noticed that the effect of magnetic field in attraction mode on inhibiting E-coli enzymatic activity was much more extensive than that in repelling mode. On the other hand, the static magnetic field of orthodontic magnets dramatically inhibits Staphylococci aurous (intraoral bacteria) growth under the two condition, attraction and repelling modes. It is observed that the effect of magnetic field in attraction mode on staphylococci aurous growth is more extensive than that in repelling mode. On the other hand, in the two types of bacteria, the dramatic effect of exposure to the static magnetic field under repelling mode covering a wider area compared to that in case of attraction mode. These significant dramatic effects were noticed after only 48 hours from exposure to the static magnetic field. Our results is in accordance with that of Bondemark et al[21] in which they concluded that; the static magnetic fields exposure values for attractive magnets were somewhat higher compared to that of repelling magnets, but the extent of the static magnetic fields is wider in case of repelling magnets compared to attracting magnets.

Short term exposure (48 hours) to the static magnetic field of orthodontic magnets in the current study; dramatically inhibit the bacterial biochemical activity and growth of E-coli and Staphylococci aurous respectively. Our findings are not in accordance with that of Bondemark et al. [16] in which they stated that “Short-term exposure to a static magnetic field did not cause any cytotoxic effect on the cells”.

In existing study it was concluded that, the static magnetic field per se could not severely affect cell growth and function the living two types of bacteria under investigation, except in the presence of trace amounts of ferrous ions. In accordance we can’t exclude the possibility of the corrosion products especially iron, released from orthodontic magnets during clinical uses, to be contributing for the observed cytotoxic effects. The conclusion of Donohue et al. [24] added more support to the combined effect of the orthodontic magnets, static magnetic field and metal ions release, they stated that their results “supports the hypothesis that these are cytotoxic effects of possibly corrosion products and of magnetism” and continued “With the evidence of a biological effect, the use of implanted magnets must at present be limited until the safety can be assured”.

The findings of Linder-Aronson et al. [25] in which they concluded that “It cannot be excluded that the magnetic field or corrosion products from the magnetic material influenced vital processes in the epithelium and the bone close to the magnets” gives more strong evidence to our findings. On the other hand Miyakoshi [26] stated that “It has also been reported that treatment with trace amounts of ferrous ions in the cell culture medium and exposure to a static magnetic field increases DNA damage, which is detected using the comet assay”.

In the current study the recorded different type of biological effects of the static magnetic field of orthodontic magnets on the cultured two types of living bacteria under investigation, in the form of growth inhibition and affecting the biochemical activity of staphylococci aurous and E-coli respectively is in accordance with that of other investigator [23] in which they stated that the effect of exposure to static magnetic fields varies depending on the cell types.

One of the most important finding of the current study is that; static magnetic field of orthodontic magnets per se had no significant effects on the cultured two types of vital cells under investigation. On the other hand, adding traces of iron to the cell culture medium enhancing the effects of static magnetic field on the different cultured cells. This result give support to the conclusion in previous clinical study by the authors in which they stated that the DNA fragmentation of the oral mucosa cells on the magnets’ side was significantly higher than that reported on the non-magnets’ side [27].

On the other hand the recorded different adverse biological effects of the static magnetic field of orthodontic magnets on one of the intraoral bacteria (Staphylococcus aurous) under investigation raised very important question of high significant clinical value. Is this means that the statistic magnetic field of orthodontic magnets could adversely affect the acquired-required balance of the intraoral flora, to the degree that it could end with intraoral pathology?! This point is in need of wide scale intensive studies.

The oral tissues, close to orthodontic magnets, are rich with blood capillaries accordingly the magnetic field will affect the oral tissues with different degrees according to distance from the orthodontic magnets, on one hand and on the other hand, the type of cells. The circulating blood in the oral tissues which are rich with iron will enhance the adverse biological effects of the static magnetic field on these tissues, even without the loss of the orthodontic magnets' protection coat. This is the critical issue in that respect! Which is in need of more intensive investigations?

The adverse biological effects of the static magnetic field of orthodontic magnets, recorded in the current study, on cell growth, function ring the bill so that orthodontic magnets should be used with great care in orthodontic practice till more complete understanding of this vital serious issue has been established.

Conclusion

The data of the current study was interpreted and discussed in view of the available literature and the following conclusions and recommendations had been extracted:

1. Exposure to static magnetic field of the commercial orthodontic samarium-cobalt (SmCo5) magnets, for only 48 hours, could adversely affect the growth and biochemical activity of vital cells.
2. The adverse biological effect of exposing Escherichia coli (E. coli) and Staphylococci aurous to the static magnetic field of orthodontic magnets fixed in attractive mode is somewhat higher compared to that of magnets fixed in repelling mode, but the extent of that destruction was wider in case of repelling magnets mode compared to that of attracting magnets mode.
3. Iron is an important factor in enhance the destructive effects of static magnetic field of orthodontic magnets on vital cells.
4. The different damaging effects of the static magnetic fields are dependent on the cell types.

References

[1] Gianelly A, Vaitas A, Thomas W. The use of magnets to move molars distally. Am. J. Orthod. Dentofac Orthop 1989; 96: 161 -7.

[2] Bondemark L, Kurol J. Distalization of maxillary first and second molars simultaneously with repelling magnets. Eur. J. Orthod. 1992; 14: 264-72.

[3] Sandler PJ. An attractive solution to unerupted teeth. Am. J. Orthod Dentofac Orthop 1991; 100: 489-93.

[4] Vardimon A, Graber TM, Drescher D, Bourauel C. Rare earth magnets and impaction. Am J Orthod Dentofac Orthop 1991; 100:494-512. Vardimon A, Graber TM, Drescher D, Bourauel C. Rare earth magnets and impaction. Am. J. Orthod. Dentofac Orthop 1991; 100:494-512.

[5] Darendeliler MA, Freidle JM. Treatment of an impacted canine with magnets. J. Clinic. Orthod 1994; 28: 639-42.

[6] Springate SD, Sandler PJ. Micro-magnetic retainer: an attractive solution to fixed retention. Br. J. Orthod 1991; 18: 139-41.

[7] Drandelier MA, Yuksel S, Meral O. Open-bite correction with magnetic activator device. *J. Clin. Orthod.* 1995; 9: 569-76.

[8] Kiliaridis S, Egermark I, Thilander B. Anterior open bite treatment with magnets. *Eur. J. Orthod.* 1990; 12:447-57.

[9] Vardimon AD, Graber TM, Voss LR, Verrusio E. Magnetic versus mechanical expansion with different force thresholds and points of application. *Am. J. Orthod. Dentofac Orthop* 1987; 92: 455-66.

[10] Vardimon AD, Graber TM, Voss LR, Muller TP. Functional orthopedic appliance (FOMA) III-Modus operandi. *Am. J. Orthod. Dentofac Orthop* 1990; 97; 135-48.

[11] Karla V, Burstone C, Nanda R. Effects of a fixed magnetic appliance on the dentofacial complex. *Am. J. Orthod Dentofac. Orthop* 1989; 95:467-78.

[12] Tsutsui H, Kinouchi Y, Sasaki H, Shiota M, Ushita T. Studies on the Sm-Co magnet as a dental material. *J. Dent Res.* 1979; 58: 1597-606.

[13] Costello J, Pratten J, Evans R, Noar J. The corrosion of rare earth orthodontic magnets. *J. Orthod* 2000; 27: 111-12.

[14] Mikloš M, Gajski G, Garaj – Vrhovac V. Usage of the standard and modified comet assay in assessment of DNA damage in human lymphocytes after exposure to ionizing radiation. *Radiol. Oncol.* 2009; 43(2): 97-107.

[15] Papadopulos M, Hoerler I, Gerber B, Rahn B, Rakosi T. Biologic effects of static magnetic fields on osteoblast cells in culture. Eur J Orthod 1990; 12: 507-21.

[16] McDonald F. Effect of static magnetic fields on osteoblasts and fibroblasts in vitro. *Bioelectromagnetics* 1993; 14: 187-96.

[17] Papadopoulos MA. Biological aspects of the use of permanent magnets and static magnetic fields in Orthodontics. *Hellenic Orthodontic Review* 1998; 1:145-57.

[18] Yamamoto Y, Ohsaki Y, Goto T, Nakasima A, Iijima T. Effects of static magnetic fields on bone formation in rat osteoblast cultures. *J. Dent Res.* 2003; 82: 962-6.

[19] Camilleri S, McDonald F. The effect of static magnetic fields on sutural cellular proliferation. *Eur. J. Orthod.* 1990; 12: 490.

[20] Camilleri S, McDonald F. Static magnetic field effect on the sagittal suture in Rattus Norvegicus. *Am. J. Orthod Dentofacial. Orthop.* 1993; 103: 240-6.

[21] Bondemark L , Kurol J, Wisten A. Extent and flux density of static magnetic fields generated by orthodontic samarium-cobalt magnets. *Am. J. Orthod. Dentofac Orthop* 1995; 107: 488-96.

[22] Miyakoshi J. The review of cellular effects of a static magnetic field. *Science and Technology of Advanced Materials*. 2006; 7: 305–307

[23] Raylman RR, Clavo AC, Wahl RL. Exposure to strong static magnetic field slows the growth of human cancer cells in vitro. *Bioelectromagnetics.* 1996; 17(5):358-63.

[24] Donohue VE, McDonald F, Evans R. In vitro cytotoxicity testing of neodymium-iron-boron magnets. *J. Appl. Biomater.* 1995; 6:69–74.

[25] Linder-Aronson S, Lindskog S. A morphometric study of bone surfaces and skin reactions after stimulation with static magnetic fields in rats. *Am. J. Orthod Dentofacial Orthop.* 1991; 99:44–8.

[26] Miyakoshi J. Effects of static magnetic fields at the cellular level. *Prog. Biophys. Mol. Biol.* 2005; 87(2-3):213-23.

[27] Abdel-Kader HM, Aref MI, Hussein FA. Coating Failure of Commercial Orthodontic Magnets and DNA Fragmentation in Oral Mucosa Cells. *AOJ* 2008: 24; 32-40.

In: A Window on Surgery and Orthodontics
Editor: Giuseppe Alessandro Scardina
ISBN: 978-1-62808-948-6

Chapter VIII

Subpedicle Connective Tissue Graft – A Bilaminar Reconstructive Surgical Procedure for Root Coverage

Prashant A. Bhusari[1] **and Manohar L. Bhongade**[2#]*
[1]Modern Dental College and Research Center, Department of Periodontics, College of Dental Surgery, Manipal, Karnataka, India
[2]Sharad Pawar Dental College and Hospital, Department of Periodontics, College of Dental Surgery, Manipal, Karnataka, India

Abstract

Background: Root coverage is the goal of periodontal plastic surgery when treating gingival recession. This article describes the use of Subpedicle Connective Tissue Graft (SPCTG) as a bilaminar reconstructive procedure for root coverage. The success of this graft has been attributed to the double blood supply at the recipient site from the underlying bone base and the overlying recipient flap.

Method: The operation SPCTG was performed on 15 sites with an isolated gingival recession accompanied by an absence of attached gingiva. The connective tissue graft was obtained from palate at premolar-molar area. All patients were evaluated at 7,15,30,60 and 90 days post-operatively.

Results: From the analysis of results, statistically highly significant root coverage was obtained at 90 days with the mean gain of 84. 66%. The mean area of gingival recession was reduced from 8. 2 $mm^2 \pm 2.$ 99 mm^2 to 1. 83 $mm^2 \pm 3.$ 11 mm^2 ($p<0.$ 001). Statistically significant increase in the width of attached gingiva was also obtained with the mean gain of 4. 6 mm. The mean width of attached gingiva was increased from o mm ±o mm to 4. 6 mm ±1. 25 mm ($p<0.$ 01).

---

* Correspondence to: Prashant A Bhusari, Address- B-102, Staff Quarters, Modern Dental College and Research Center, Gandhinagar, P.O Box-453112, Indore, Madhya Pradesh, India. Email- pbhu2000use@yahoo.co.in. Fax- 0091-0731-2882699, 0091-0731-2882700.

This study was supported by College of Dental Surgery, Manipal.

Conclusions: Based on the results, the SPCTG technique showed high predictability in the treatment of single recession.

Keywords: Periodontal surgery; gingival; recession; root coverage; grafts

Introduction

Periodontics has long has been concerned with commonly occurring problems of isolated gingival recession and root exposure. In addition to the esthetic concern of a patient, exposed root surfaces are frequently associated with hypersensitivity and plaque retention. When the recession extends to or through mucogingival line, it causes a break in the continuity of the attached gingiva and a localized shallowing of vestibular fornix. In these circumstances further recession may be contributed to or promoted by the adverse pull of the facial musculature on the most apical tissue of the lesion.

Even though etiology of gingival recession still needs elucidation, several techniques have been proposed to treat it like lateral pedicle graft (LPG) [1], free gingival graft (FGG) [2], semilunar coronally positioned flap (SCPF) [3], connective tissue graft (CTG) [4],coronally advanced flap (CAF) [5], coronally advanced flap with connective tissue graft (CAF+CTG) [6], coronally advanced flap with acellular dermal matrix (CAF+ADM)[7]. In addition various regenerative procedures such as the use of non-resorbable barriers, bioresorbable barriers (GTR) [8], enamel matrix derivative (EMD) [9] and the application of platelet rich plasma (PRP) [10] in combination with coronally advanced flap are also used to treat gingival recessions.

Although these techniques have shown a consistent potential for root coverage, meta analysis from several systematic reviews revealed an ample degree of variability of clinical results [11, 12, 13]. The outcome of these reviews showed a greater recession reduction and a large amount of root completely covered following bilaminar techniques (CAF+CTG) as compared with regenerative procedures. The introduction of guided tissue regeneration (GTR) in the treatment of gingival recession allowed clinician to avoid a second surgical site and to achieve a predictable new connective tissue attachment over the exposed root surface[8]. But the controlled clinical trials have indicated that GTR based root coverage procedures reported well especially in deep and narrow defects [14]. More recently EMD was used in combination with coronally advanced flap, resulting in improved outcome with combined approach [9]. A randomized controlled study compared CAF+EMD versus CAF+CTG [15]. Authors reported that the latter resulted in greater increase in height of keratinized tissue at 24 months but there was no difference in terms of root coverage. An ADM has also been recently proposed as a replacement for CTG in bilaminar techniques with promising clinical outcomes in terms of root coverage [16].

The bilaminar techniques are actually perceived as the most reliable procedure. It has also been clinically demonstrated that Sub Pedicle Connective Tissue Graft (SPCTG) yields results producing better healing and less operative discomfort at the donor site when compared to free gingival graft. It also offers a dual blood supply, a better color match and a high degree of predictable success [11].

In the light of increasing knowledge on reconstructive mucogingival surgery for coverage of gingival recession, the present study was therefore an attempt to evaluate biometrically the predictability of Subpedicle Connective Tissue Graft as described by Nelson [17], to cover the denuded root surface.

Materials and Methods

A total of fifteen patients, eleven male and four females were selected from the outpatient department of College Of Dental Surgery Manipal, Karnataka, India. Their age varied from 18 to 35 years. All the patients were periodontally and systemically healthy with no contraindication for periodontal surgery. All of them were non-smoker and had not taken medications known to interfere with periodontal tissue health or healing.

The criteria for inclusion in the study was the presence of localized gingival recession with minimal or no attached gingiva irrespective of the width and length of recession or position of the affected teeth in the arch. In addition there was no loss of interdental bone on radiograph.

Initial Therapy: All the patients received scaling, curettage and root planning prior to surgical therapy. The teeth with prominent root convexities were planed excessively to reduce the convexities. Occlusal premature contacts were checked and eliminated by using articulating paper and grinding stones. A thorough plaque control programme was initiated for each patient including instructions in brushing technique and supervised teeth brushing. The patients selected were informed of the treatment options and written consent received from all the patients.

A week after initial preparation, the patients were reexamined in order to ascertain the periodontal status of each patient. The degree of gingival inflammation was monitored by using Gingival Index, a component of Periodontal Disease Index. (Ramfjord 1959) Oral hygiene effectiveness was monitored by Quigley- Hein Plaque Index (1970), since patients were required to achieve plaque control success at or below the 10% of efficiency before surgical therapy was initiated.

Clinical Parameters: Prior to surgery following measurements were taken using cemento-enamel junction as a fixed point.

1. Cemento-enamel junction to gingival margin = Recession depth (RD)
2. Gingival margin to base of sulcus = Probing depth (PD)
3. Gingival margin to mucogingival junction = Width of keratinized gingival (WKG)
4. Width of gingival recession at cement-enamel junction = (RW)
5. Width of attached gingival = WKG-PD
6. Area of gingival recession = ½ RD x RW

These measurements were made at midfacial surface of the tooth to be treated with the help of William's Periodontal Probe to the nearest millimeter. Teeth adjacent to the area of gingival recession either had no clinical recession or a lesser amount, were used as a donor or control teeth. Measurements were also recorded on control teeth.

Surgical Procedure

Recipient Site: One hour prior to surgery oral antibiotic (Cap Tetracycline 250 mg) was commenced and continued at the rate of 1gm/day for 5 days with non-narcotic analgesic containing “Analgin” as a main ingredient. An antiseptic solution. ” Mercury Chrome” was applied on the field of operation with cotton swab. The area was anesthetized using 2% xylocaine with 1:50,000 epinephrine on both the facial and lingual aspect. After sometime anesthesia was tested by subjective and objective test.

Preparation of recipient site was initiated with two vertical incisions made from the proximal line angles of adjacent teeth at the level of cement-enamel junction to the base of the vestibule with No. 15 Bard-Parker blade. These incisions were horizontally connected to the internal bevel incision that was made 1mm parallel to the border of the recession and U shaped collar of the gingival was removed. A full-thickness mucogingival flap was reflected with periosteal elevator to allow repositioning of pedicle to the cement-enamel junction of the affected tooth. The root was reinspected to assure that all roughness had been removed and covered with moist gauze.

Donor Site: After anesthetizing the gingival zone of palate near premolar-molar area, incisions were made by No. 15 Bard Parker blade in palate following the outline of tinfoil template. Perpendicular incisions were made to establish the correct width of graft. A partial thickness flap was reflected and cut to expose the underlying connective tissue. The connective tissue graft was separated from the underlying tissue by sharp dissection and was detached at its base by a horizontal incision. After removal, the graft was examined for glandular/fatty tissue, surface irregularities and thickness. Correction of all these properties was done with scalpel blade or scissors while graft was held in gauze moistened with normal saline solution. To minimize trauma and dehydration graft was placed on a previously prepared recipient bed as soon as possible.

Stabilization of Graft on Recipient Bed

The connective tissue graft which was placed on the recipient bed at the level of cement-enamel junction was sutured to the adjacent coronal margins of interdental papillae with 5-0 plain resorbable sutures. Slight firm pressure with saline soaked gauze was maintained until initial clotting occurred, providing some fixation for the graft and avoiding the dead space under the graft tissue.

Acromycin ointment 3% (Tetracyclin HCL) was applied on sutures. Following placement of free connective tissue graft, the pedicle flap was positioned as a Double Papillae Pedicle Graft directly over that part of connective tissue graft that was overlying the denuded root surface and sutured by sling suture. Again the Acromycin ointment was applied on the sutures and pedicle graft. The recipient area was then covered with tinfoil to prevent incorporation of sutures into the periodontal dressing (Coe-pack). The periodontal dressing was placed over the recipient and donor site.

Post Surgical Care

The periodontal dressing and the sutures were removed after one week and wound cleaned with 3% Hydrogen Peroxide solution. The periodontal dressing was then placed and again removed after two weeks. The teeth were polished with polishing paste and rubber cup. The patients were instructed in oral hygiene.

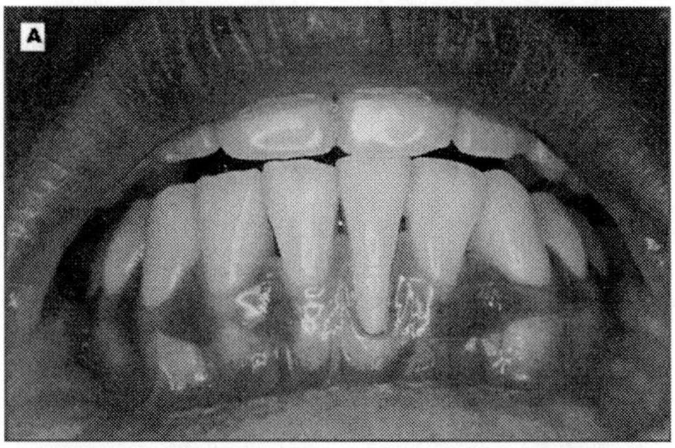

A) Preoperative clinical view of gingival recession.

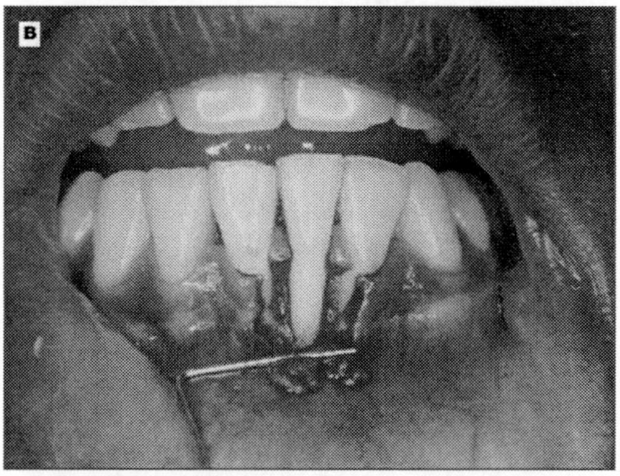

B) Double papillae reflected from donor site.

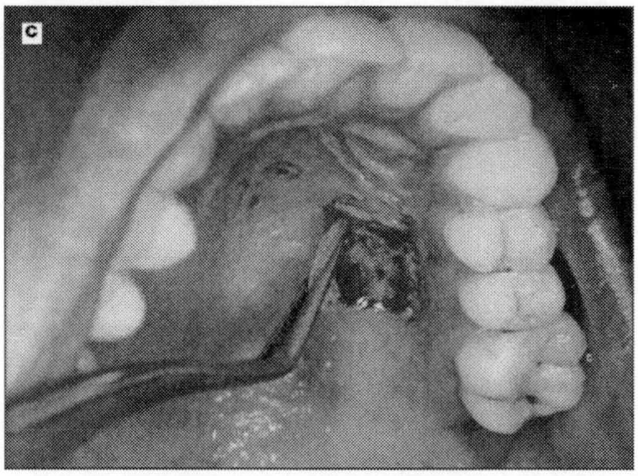

C) Split thickness flap reflected from donor site.

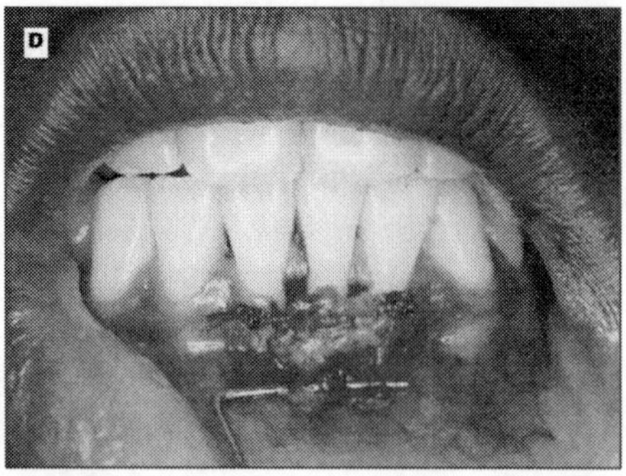

D) Connective tissue graft sutured on the recipient site.

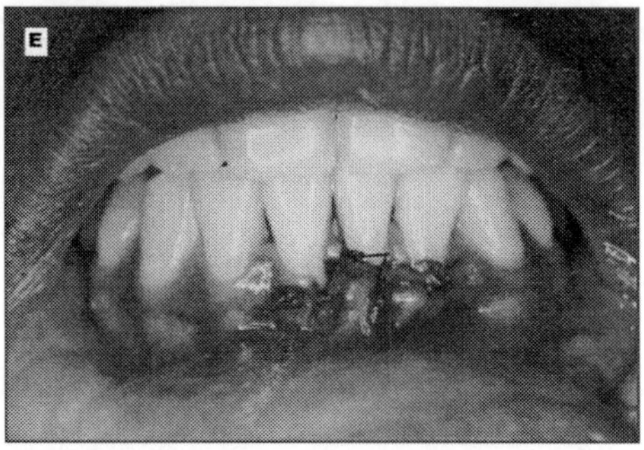

E) Double papillae graft sutured over connective tissue graft.

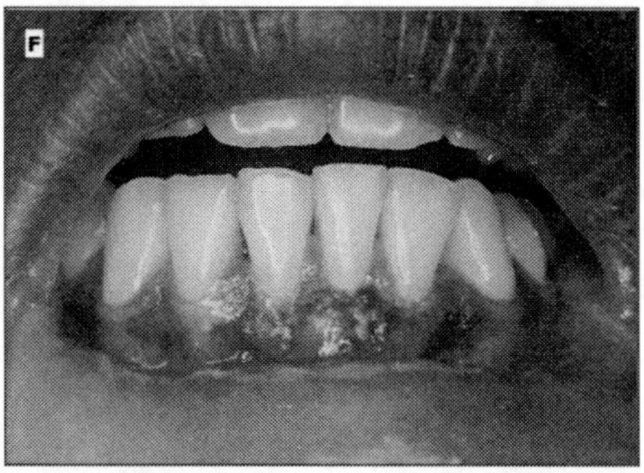

F) 7 days after treatment.

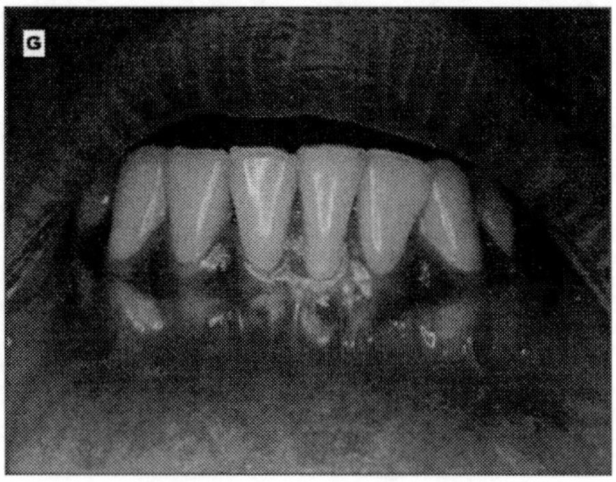

G) 60 days after treatment.

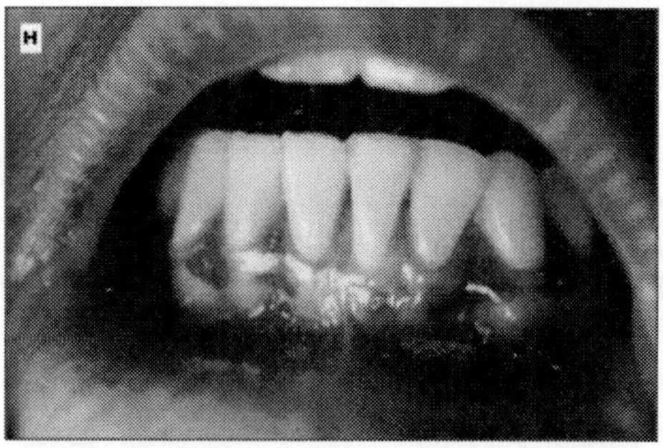

H) 90 days after treatment.

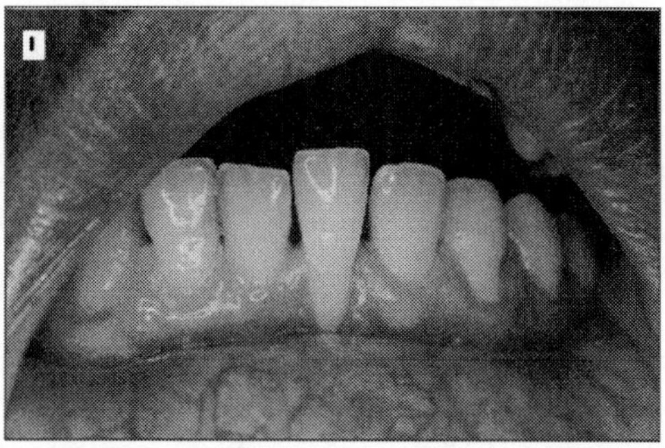

I) Preoperative clinical view of gingival recession.

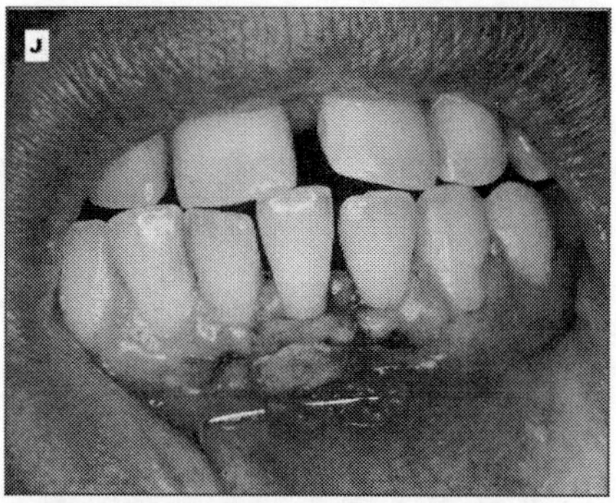

J) Double papillae graft reflected from donor site.

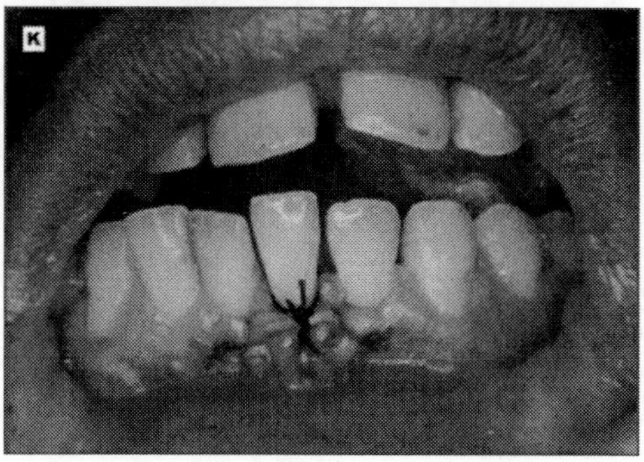

K) Connective tissue graft sutured on the recipient area.

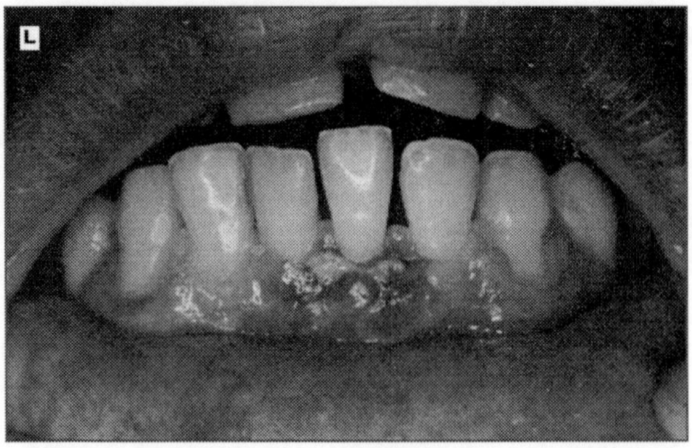

L) Double papillae graft sutured over connective tissue graft.

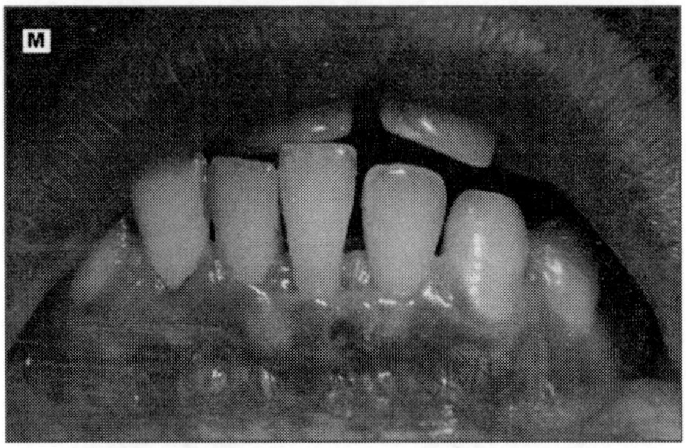

M) 90 days after treatment.

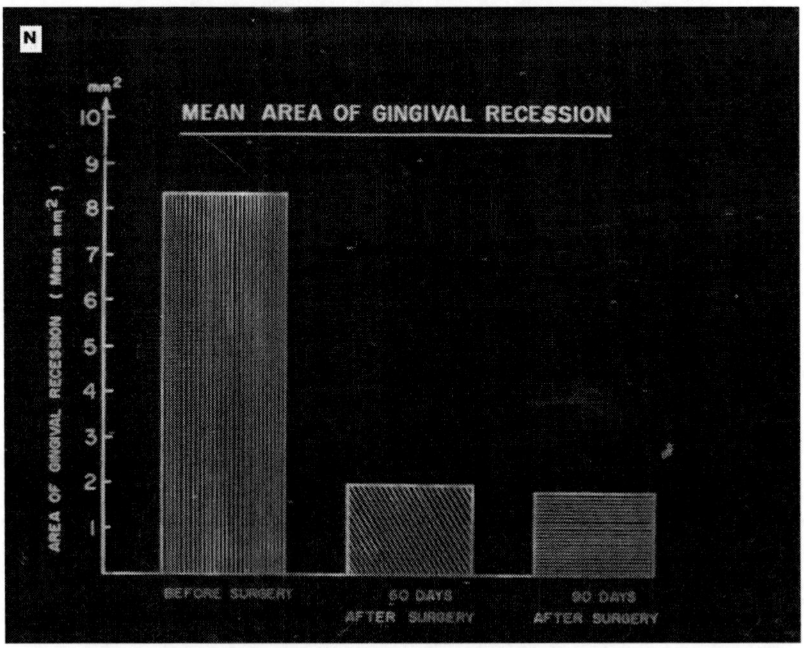

N) Histogram illustrating area of gingival recession.

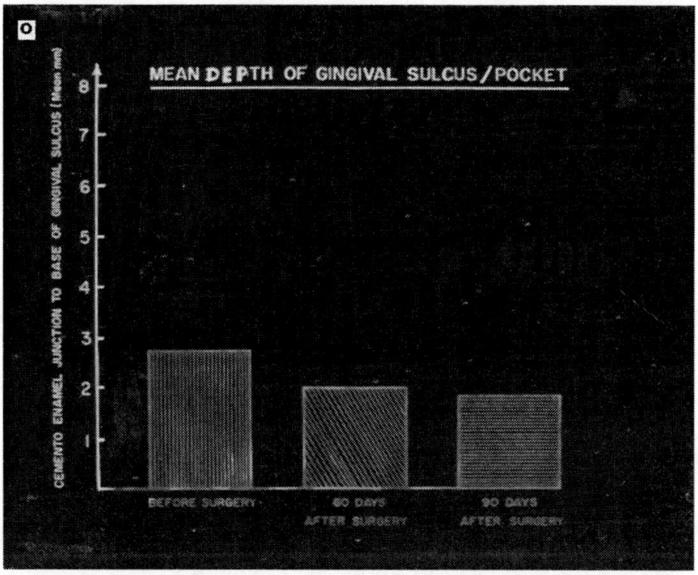

O) Histogram illustrating mean depth of gingival sulcus before and after surgery.

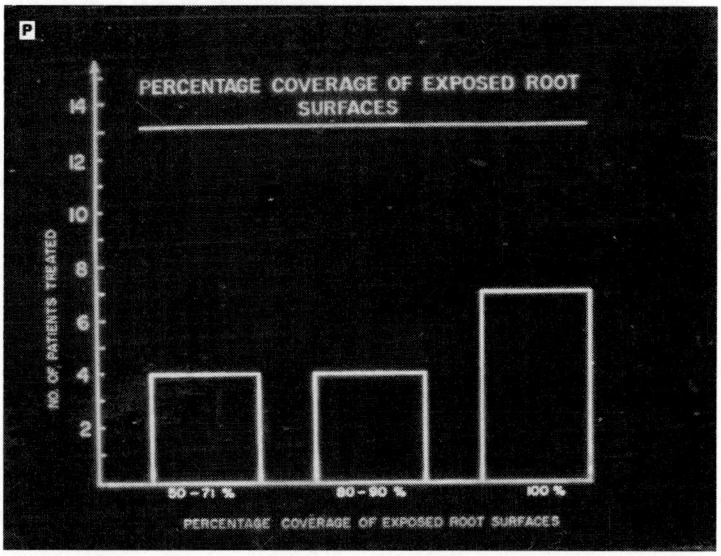

P) Histogram illustrating percentages of root coverage after 90 days.

Statistical Analysis

All preoperative measurements were repeated postsurgically at 7, 15, 30, 60 and 90 days except sulcus depths which were measured at 60 and 90 days postsurgically. The photographs were taken pre and post operatively to provide an indication of changes in color and contour. All data obtained were analyzed biometrically using Paired “t” test to determine the significance of results.

Results

In this study, a total of 15 sites (in 15 patients) with gingival recession ranging from 3 mm to 12 mm (area of gingival recession ranging from 4 mm^2 to 30 mm^2) were treated by SPCTG. In order to minimize the variations in surgical technique, all procedures were completed by one surgeon, who also followed up the patients for a period of 3 months. All the grafts appeared successful take and no complication of infection e. g.: pain, bleeding, suppuration, swelling nor discomfort was reported by any of the patients during the healing period. The preoperative (at baseline) and postoperative (at 60 and 90 days) reading of sulcus/pocket depth, root coverage, width of keratinized tissue and width of attached gingiva were tabulated (Table 1 and 2). The results were subjected to statistical analysis using paired "t" test (Table 3 and 4). The results were considered significant and highly significant when p< 0. 01 and p< 0. 001 respectively.

Table 1. Dimensions of gingival recession (width and length) on recipient teeth before surgery and length of gingival recession after surgery

Case	Tooth no.	Preoperative recession		Recession length after root coverage						
		Length	Width	Immediately after operation	07 days	15 days	30 days	60 days	90 days	
		mm	mm	mm	mm	mm	mm	mm	mm	%
01	24	4	3	0	2	2	2	2	2	50
02	25	4	3	0	0	0	0	0	0	100
03	25	4	2	0	0	0	0	0	0	100
04	24	5	3	0	0	0	1	1	1	80
05	24	3	3	0	0	0	0	0	0	100
06	5	4	3	0	1	1	1	1	0	100
07	25	5	3	0	0	0	0	0	0	100
08	24	6	3	0	0	0	1	1	1	83. 33
09	24	5	3	0	0	0	2	2	2	60
10	25	5	2	0	0	0	0	0	0	100
11	25	7	3	0	3	3	3	3	2	71. 42
12	6	5	3	0	0	0	1	1	1	86. 66
13	24	3	3	0	0	0	0	0	0	100
14	25	5	3	0	0	0	1	1	1	80
15	6	12	5	0	5	5	5	5	5	56. 66
Mean										84. 66

The depth of gingival sulcus/pocket was compared pre and post operatively but there was little difference in the mean values over 3 months period. The mean preoperative sulcus depth was 2. 7 mm±1. 53 mm with the range of 2 to 8 mm which was improved to 2. 06 mm ± 0. 27

mm after 60 days and 2. 06 mm ±1 mm after 90 days. The mean difference of 0. 6 mm and 0. 66 mm was found to be statistically less significant ($p<0.05$). Out of 15 sites, 7 showed 100% root coverage, 4 sites showed root coverage between 50 to 70% and 4 sites showed root coverage between 80 to 90%.

The mean area of root coverage obtained at the end of 90 days was 84. 66%. Preoperatively mean area of gingival recession was 8. 2 mm^2 ± 2. 99 mm^2 with the range of 4 to 30 mm^2 which improved to 2. 03 mm^2 ±3. 20 mm^2 after 60 days and 1. 83 mm^2 ± 3. 11 mm^2 after 90 days. The mean difference of 6. 16 mm^2 and 6. 36 mm^2 was found to be statistically highly significant ($p<0.001$). Preoperatively the mean width of keratinized gingiva was 1. 6 mm ±1. 12 mm with a range of 0 to 3 mm. The mean width of keratinized gingiva was improved to 6. 4 mm ± 1mm after 60 days and 6. 6 mm ±1. 19 mm after 90 days. The mean difference of 4. 8 mm and 4. 9 mm was found to be statistically highly significant ($p<0.001$).

Preoperatively the mean width of attached gingiva was 0 mm ± 0 mm which was improved to 4. 3 mm ± 1 mm after 60 days and 4. 6 mm ±1. 25 mm after 90 days. The mean difference of 4. 3 mm and 4. 5 mm was found to be statistically highly significant ($p<0.001$).

Table 2. Width of keratinized gingival, gingival sulcus depth and width of attached gingival on recipient site before and after surgery

Case	Tooth no.	Keratinized gingiva GM – MGJ (mm)			Gingival sulcus / pocket depth (mm)									Attached gingiva (mm) Keratinized gingival – gingiva sulcus / pocket depth		
		Pre operative	60 days	90 days	Pre-operative			Post-operative						Pre-operative	60 days	90 days
								60 days			90 days					
					M	B	D	M	B	D	M	B	D			
01	24	3	7	7	2	3	2	2	3	3	2	2	3	0	5	5
02	25	2	6	6	2	2	3	2	2	2	2	2	2	0	4	4
03	25	3	7	7	3	2	3	2	2	2	2	2	2	0	5	5
04	24	2	8	8	2	2	3	2	2	2	2	2	2	0	6	6
05	24	2	7	8	3	3	3	2	2	3	2	2	3	0	5	6
06	5	1	7	8	3	2	3	3	2	2	2	2	2	0	5	6
07	25	2	7	8	2	2	2	2	2	3	2	2	3	0	5	6
08	24	0	6	6	3	3	3	2	2	2	2	2	2	0	4	4
09	24	2	5	5	3	2	3	2	2	3	2	2	2	0	3	3
10	25	2	6	6	2	2	2	2	2	2	2	2	2	0	4	4
11	25	0	4	4	3	2	3	2	2	2	2	2	2	0	2	2
12	06	3	7	7	2	3	3	3	2	3	3	2	3	0	5	5
13	24	2	6	6	3	2	3	2	2	3	2	2	3	0	4	4
14	25	0	6	6	3	2	3	2	2	3	2	2	2	0	4	4
15	6	0	7	7	3	8	3	2	3	2	2	3	2	0	4	4
Mean		1. 6	6. 4	6. 6	2. 6	2. 7	2. 8	2. 1	2. 06	2. 4	2. 0	2. 06	2. 3	0. 0	4. 6	4. 53

GM: Gingival Margin.

Table 3. Statistical analysis of results on recipient teeth after 60 days

S. No.	Parameters	Before surgery n=15		60 days after surgery n=15						
		Mean	S. D.	Mean	S. D.	Mean diff.	S. D. diff	t value	p value	Statistical analysis
1	Gingival sulcus depth (mm)	2. 7	1. 53	2. 06	0. 27	0. 6	1. 29	1. 739	p < . 05	Less significant
2	Gingival recession (mm)	8. 2	2. 99	2. 03	3. 20	6. 16	3. 35	6. 877	p < . 001	Highly significant
3	Keratinized gingiva (mm)	1. 6	1. 12	7. 4	1. 00	4. 8	1. 14	14. 74	p < . 001	Highly significant
4	Attached gingiva (mm)	0	0	4. 3	1. 00	4. 3	0. 97	16. 57	p < . 001	Highly significant

Table 4. Statistical analysis of results on recipient teeth after 90 days

S. No.	Parameters	Before surgery n=15		90 days after surgery n=15						
		Mean	S. D.	Mean	S. D.	Mean diff.	S. D. diff	t value	p value	Statistical analysis
1	Gingival sulcus depth (mm)	2. 7	1. 53	2. 06	1. 00	0. 66	1. 28	1. 92	p < . 05	Less significant
2	Gingival recession (mm)	8. 2	2. 99	1. 83	3. 11	6. 36	3. 57	6. 66	p < . 001	Highly significant
3	Keratinized gingiva (mm)	1. 6	1. 121	6. 6	1. 19	4. 9	1. 27	14. 42	p < . 001	Highly significant
4	Attached gingiva (mm)	0	0	4. 6	1. 25	4. 5	1. 72	3. 78	p < . 001	Significant

The depth of gingival sulcus, area of gingival recession, width of keratinized gingival and attached gingival were compared pre and postoperatively on donor teeth but there was little difference in their mean values during 3 months of observation period. The mean preoperative sulcus depth, at the mid facial surface of donor teeth (neighbouring to the treated teeth) were 2. 6mm and 2. 8 mm; with the range of 2 to 3 mm. After 90 days the mean sulcus depth was 2. 06mm and 2. 06 mm. The mean difference was very little and the result was not statistically significant. The mean preoperative areas of gingival recession were 0. 3mm^2 and 0. 13 mm^2 with the range of 0 to 3 mm^2. The mean areas of gingival recession at 90 days were 0. 2mm^2 and 0. 4mm^2 with negligible difference. The mean preoperative width of gingiva was 5. 2mm and 5 mm on either side of recipient teeth with the range of 3 to 6 mm. 90 days postoperatively the mean width of gingiva was 5 mm and 4. 8 mm with the mean difference of 0. 2mm and 0. 3 mm. The mean preoperative widths of attached gingiva were 2. 9mm and 2. 6 mm on the donor teeth adjacent to the recipient area. 90 days post operatively the mean width of attached gingiva was 3 mm and 2. 7 mm with negligible difference.

Discussion

Obtaining predictable root coverage becomes an important part of periodontal therapy. Many different types of surgical procedures have been used to achieve root coverage but produced unsatisfactory results [1-10]. There are many reasons for these failures. They include: poor case selection, improper technique selection, unrealistic goals and lack of experience in performing reconstructive periodontal plastic procedures.

Of the various techniques used, SPCTG is considered the gold standard treatment for coverage of denuded roots. In this study during preparation of recipient bed, a full thickness flap was reflected for the following reasons: 1)Attempt made to prevent bone loss by reflecting a partial thickness flap, may sometimes result in flap perforation which in turn can lead to flap necrosis and further bone loss [18]. 2) With full thickness flap/SPCTG, rapid capillary proliferation from the periosteal surface of the full thickness flap approximating the outer surface of the connective tissue graft is anticipated [19]. 3) Also highly vascularized tissue adjacent to a root surface (as in case of partial thickness flap) has been suggested as a necessary condition for root resorption. Hence Periodontist performing partial thickness connective tissue graft should be alert to the possible occurrence of external root resorption over extended period of time [20]. Full thickness flap/SPCTG has been studied in detail by many workers [17, 19, 21].

Root preparation before root coverage can be mechanical, chemical or combination of both. Owing to the risk and limited benefit of root demineralization with chemical agents [22], in the present study, root preparation was limited to mechanical scaling and root planing.

In this study, a total of 15 sites with gingival recession ranging from 3 mm to 12 mm were treated with SPCTG. The patients were followed for up to 3 months. Zingale [23] and Egli [24] et al. reported no significant variation in the amount of root coverage between 1 and 12 months observation period. The stability of their results after 30 days were observed both on recipient as well as on the donor teeth for all variables tested. Therefore 3 months postoperative examination permitted us an evaluation of predictability of results for the SPCTG technique.

Orientation of the superficial surface of the CTG was not specific to either the gingival flap or the root surface. This is in accordance with the study done by Mohammad et al. [25], which indicated that the surface orientation of the CTG had no significant effect on the clinical outcome of root coverage. After placing the procured graft over the recipient bed, it was covered by coronally positioned double papillary pedicle flap. A recent study [26] concluded that the more coronal the level of gingival margin after suturing, the greater the probability of complete root coverage. Accordingly, in this study, the flap covered the graft as much as possible and was coronally positioned and sutured.

With SPCTG, the mean root coverage obtained in the present study at the end of 3 months was 84. 53%. This coverage of denuded root surface was statistically significant. This was found to be well within the limits of the studies done by Broghetti et al. [21] and Harris et al. [27] who obtained root coverage of 70. 5% and 97. 6% respectively.

The root coverage obtained with this bilaminar technique was found to be less than that obtained by Tozum et al. [28] (96. 4%) who used the pouch and tunnel technique with SCTG for root coverage. The increased percentage of root coverage obtained in this study may be due to minimal incisions and reflection of the flap allowing unhindered blood supply. This technique is especially effective for the maxillary anterior area where vestibular depth is adequate and there is good gingival thickness [29]. In contrast in the present study maxillary premolars and advanced gingival recessions were also included.

Out of 15 sites, 7 sites showed 100% root coverage, 4 sites showed 50 to 70 % root coverage and 4 sites showed 80 to 90% root coverage. Complete root coverage was obtained in 46. 62% of the sites and it was correlated well with the study by Paolantonio et al. [30], who observed complete root coverage in 46. 6% of the sites treated with SPCTG. The mean area of gingival recession reduction of 6. 36 mm^2 obtained in this study is comparable with the results obtained by Borghetti et al. [31] and Carvalho de Silva et al. [32].

Modification of the apico-coronal dimensions of the mucogingival complex appears to be common following periodontal plastic surgery. Several surgical procedures have been proposed and practiced to increase the width of keratinized gingival tissue in order to assist proper plaque control and prevent further recession of the gingival margin.

In the present study there is an increase in the width of keratinized gingiva from baseline to the third month; from 1. 6 mm ±1. 12 to 6. 6 mm ±1. 19 mm. The mean gain in the width of keratinized gingiva at the end of 3 months was 4. 9 mm which was statistically highly significant (p<0. 001) and correlates well with the studies done by Borghetti et al. [31] and Harris et al. [27]. It is commonly believed that CTG would contribute to keratinization of the overlying epithelium.

The mean pocket depth reduction of 0. 6 mm from the base line is statistically less significant (p<0. 005). The results obtained in the present study are consistent with the studies done by Paolantonio et al. [30] and Carvalho De Silva et al. [32]. Clinically it was difficult to penetrate the sulcus with a probe. There was no bleeding on probing. These findings were compatible with a healthy attachment. SCTG yielded excellent color and tissue blending. Not a single patient had enlarged marginal gingiva and required gingivoplasty.

Although the bilaminar technique using SCTG still holds the most promising results in root coverage, histologic studies show unpredictable healing regeneration, if any, is found at the most apical portion [14]. This has encouraged investigations on techniques of a more regenerative nature.

The use of barrier membranes either resorbable or non-resorbable in the procedure of GTR is an important trend in regenerating the lost periodontal structures in periodontitis. In general, the percentage of root coverage obtained in GTR ranges from 45% to 92% [33]. The results of the present study are also within the range of root coverage obtained by barrier membranes (45% to 92%). Muller et al. [34] demonstrated only 50% coverage of recession when applying a bioresorbable membrane in shallow defects, They concluded that shallow recession should not be treated with GTR.

The purpose of developing newer and newer techniques of root coverage is to increase predictability, reduce patient discomfort and number of surgical sites and to satisfy the patient's esthetic demands. Acellular Dermal Matrix (ADM) [16] graft is a human soft tissue chemically procured to remove all epithelial and dermal cells (antigenic cells) while preserving the remaining bioactive dermal matrix composed of collagen, elastin, blood vessels. This supports vascularization, cell proliferation and tissue remodeling which facilitates its integration into the periodontal tissue. Sites treated with ADM had mean root coverage of 89. 14 %(ranged from 83. 3% to 95. 8%) [35] which is similar to the percentage of root coverage obtained in the present study. Reported disadvantages of ADM were postoperative discomfort and cost effectiveness. Postoperative discomfort may be attributed to the initial reaction of the body to a foreign grafting material.

The use of enamel matrix protein is one trend aiming at periodontal regeneration and root coverage. Hagewald et al. [36] found 2. 9 mm of recession reduction with 80% of root coverage 12 months after therapy. The results of the present study are comparable to the results obtained by Hagewald et al.

Evidence suggests that platelet rich plasma (PRP) has potential to enhance periodontal regeneration. As platelet concentrate has higher concentrate of platelet per milli-liter, it may contain higher concentration of growth factors to accelerate or enhance regeneration. PRP has been shown to enhance soft tissue healing, promote initial stabilization and revascularization of the flap and grafts in the root coverage procedures [37]. Termee J Griffin et al. [38] reported 2 cases of gingival recession treated by coronally positioned flap with platelet concentrate graft. They obtained complete root coverage in both the cases with gain of 1. 5 mm of keratinized tissue in one case. The techniques to produce PRP are found to be very sensitive and require a learning curve. Sometimes a very small volume of PRP may be procured from whole blood. So preparation techniques also contribute to the variations in the volume of PRP and eventually the percentage of root coverage.

Recent evidence [13] also suggests that among all the plastic surgical procedures for root coverage, SPCTG remains the most effective.

Within its limitations, the results of this study demonstrated that SPCTG is an effective technique to obtain root coverage.

Conclusion

The following conclusions can be made from the present study:

1. SPCTG is a safe and effective method for the treatment of gingival recession.
2. Statistically significant root coverage of 84. 66% was obtained by this surgical procedure.
3. The root coverage obtained improved the esthetic and met the expectations and demands of the patients as well as of the treating surgeon.
4. No complications were encountered in any patients who participated in this study.

The results should be interpreted with due consideration given to the relatively small sample size (n=15) and the short evaluation period (3 months).

Acknowledgments

This study was supported by College of Dental Surgery, Manipal, Karnataka, India. The authors report no conflict of interest related to this study.

References

[1] Grupe H, Warren RJ. Repair of gingival defects by a sliding flap operation. *J. Periodontol* 1956; 27:290-295.

[2] Brackett RC, Gargiulo AW. Free gingival grafts in humans. J. Periodontol 1970; 41:581.

[3] Tarnow DP. Semilunar coronally repositioned flap. *J. Clinical Periodontol* 1986; 13:182.

[4] Levine RA. Covering denuded root surface with the sub epithelial connective tissue graft. *Compend Contin Educ Dent* 1991; 12:568.

[5] Harvery PM. Management of advanced periodontitis. I. Preliminary report of a method of surgical reconstruction. *NZ Dent. J.* 1965; 61:180-187.

[6] Langer B, Langer L. Sub epithelial connective tissue graft technique for root coverage. *J. Periodontol* 1985; 56:715-20.

[7] Harris RJ. A short term and long term comparison of root coverage with an Acellular dermal matrix and a sub epithelial graft. *J. Periodontol* 2005; 75:734-743.

[8] Tatakis DN and Trombellil. Gingival recession treatment: guided tissue regeneration with bioresorbable membrane versus connective tissue graft. *J. Periodontol* 2000; 71:299-307.

[9] Spahr A, Hagewald S, Tsoulfidou F, Rompola E, and Heijl L. Coverage of Miller class I and II recession defect using enamel matrix proteins versus coronally advanced flap technique: a two year report. *J. Periodontol* 2005; 76:1871-1880.

[10] Lien-Hai Huang, Rodrigo EF Neiva, Stephen E, Soehren, William V Giannobile et al. The effect of platelet rich plasma on the coronally advanced flap root coverage procedure: a pilot human trial. *J. Periodontol* 2005; 76:1768-1777.

[11] Roccuzzo M, Bunino M, Needleman I and Senz M. Periodontal plastic surgery for treatment of localized gingival recession: a systematic review. *J. Clinical Periodontol* 2002; 29 (suppl. 3), 178-194.

[12] Clauser C, Nierim M, Franceschi D, Pagliaro V and Pini Prato. Evidence based mucogingival therapy. Part II: ordinary and indivisual patient data meta analysis of surgical treatment of recession using complete root coverage as the outcome variable. *J. Periodontol* 2003; 74:741-756.

[13] Cairo F, Pagliaro V and Nieri M. Treatment of gingival recession with coronally advanced flap procedures. A systematic review. *J. Clinical Periodontology* 2008; 35 (suppl.): 141-167.

[14] Majzoab Z, Landi L, Grusovin MG, Cardioli G. Histology of connective tissue graft. A case report. *J. Periodontol* 2001; 1607-1615.

[15] MC Guire MK and Nunn M. Evaluation of human recession defects treated with coronally advanced flaps and either enamel matrix derivative or connective tissue. Past I: comparison of clinical parameters. *J. Periodontol* 2003; 74:1110-1125.

[16] Harris R. A comparative study of root coverage obtained with an acellular dermal matrix versus a connective tissue graft: results of 107 recession defects in 50 consecutively treated patients. *2000 International Journal of Periodontics and Restorative Dentistry*, 20: 51-59.

[17] Nelson S. The Subpedicle connective tissue graft, a bilaminar reconstructive procedure for the coverage of denuded root surfaces. *J. Periodontol* 1987; 58:95-102.

[18] Staflileno H, significant differences and advantages between the full thickness and split thickness flaps. 1974; *J. Periodontol*; 45:421-5.

[19] Wilcko MT, Wilcko WM, Murphy KG, Carroll WJ, Ferguson DJ, Miley DD et al. Full thickness flap/Sub epithelial connective tissue, grafting with intramarrow penetration: three case reports of lingual root coverage. *Int J. Periodontics Restorative dent* 2005; 25:561-9.

[20] Hokett SD, Peacock ME, Burns WT, Swiec GD, Cuenin MF. External Root Resorption following partial thickness connective tissue placement: A case report. *J. Periodontol* 2002; 73:334-9.

[21] Borghetti A, Louise F. Controlled clinical evaluation of the sub pedicle connective tissue graft for the coverage of gingival recession. *J. Periodontol* 1194; 65:1107-12.

[22] Caffesse RG, La Rossa M, Garza M, Travers AM, Mondragon J, Weltman R. Citric acid demineralization and sub pedicle connective tissue graft. *J. Periodontol* 2000; 71: 568 -72.

[23] Zingale J. Observation on free gingival autografts. J. Periodontol 1974;45: 748.

[24] Egli U, Vollmer WH and Rateitschak KH. Follow up studies of free gingival grafts. *J. Periodontol* 1975; 2:98.

[25] Mohammed S, Nabli FB, Anthony JF, Benton Cole. Effect of connective tissue graft orientation on root coverage and gingival augmentation. *Int J. Periodont Restorative Dent* 2004; 24:65-9.

[26] Pini Prato GP, Baldi C, Nieri M, Franseschi D, Cortelleni P, Clouser C et al. Coronally advanced flap: The post surgical position of gingival margin is an important factor for achieving complete root coverage. *J. Periodontol* 2005; 76:713-22.

[27] Harris RJ. Connective tissue graft combined with either double pedicle graft or coronally positioned pedicle graft: Results of 266 consecutively treated defects in 200 patients. *Int. J. Periodont Restorative Dent* 2002; 22:463-71.

[28] Tozum TF, Keceli HG, Gencu GN, Hatipoglu H, Sengum D. Treatment of gingival recession. Comparison of two techniques of subepithelial connective tissue graft. *J. Periodontol* 2005; 76:1842-8.

[29] Newman MG, Takei HH, Klokkevold PR, Carranza FA. *Carranza's clinical periodontology* 10th ed. Elseviers Publishers: 2006, p. 1022.

[30] Paolantonio M, Dolci M, Esposito P, Archivio D, Lisanti L, Diluccio A, et al. Subpedicle Acellular dermal matrix graft and autogenous connective tissue graft in the treatment of gingival recession: A comparative one year clinical study. *J. Periodontol* 2002; 73:1299-307.

[31] Borghetti A, Glise JM Virgine MC, Jacques D. A comparative clinical study of bioresorbable membrane and SCTG in the treatment of human gingival recession. *J. Periodontol* 1999; 70:123-30.

[32] Carvallo da Silva R, Jolly JC, Martorelli de Lima AF, Tatakis DN. Root coverage using the coronally positioned flap with or without a subepithelial connective tissue graft. *J. Periodontol* 2004; 75:413-9.

[33] Harris RJ. A comparison of 2 roots coverage techniques. Guided tissue regeneration with a biodegradable matrix. Style membrane versus a connective tissue graft combined

with coronally positioned pedicle graft without vertical incisions. Results of series of consecutive causes. *J. Periodontol* 1998; 69:1426-1434.

[34] Muller HP, Stahl M. Eger T. Failure of root coverage of shallow gingival recessions employing GTE and a bioresorbable membrane. *Int J. Periodontics Restorative Dent* 2001; 171-181.

[35] Aichle mann- Reidy MB, Yokna RA, Evans GH, Nasr HF, Mayer ET. Clinical evaluation of Acellular allograft dermis for the treatment of human gingival recession. *J. Periodontol* 2002; 72:998-1005.

[36] Hagewald S, Spahr A, Rompola E, Haller B, Heijl L, Bernimoulin JP. Comparative study Emdogain and coronally advanced flop technique in the treatment of human gingival recession. A prospective controlled clinical study. *J. Clinical Periodontol* 2002; 29:35-41.

[37] Petrungaro PS. using platelet rich plasma to accelerate soft tissue maturation in esthetic periodontal surgery. *Compend Contin Dent* 2001; 22:729,732,734,736.

[38] Terrence J Griffin, Wai S. Cheung. Treatment of gingival recession with platelet concentrate graft; A report of two cases. *Int J. Periodontics Restorative Dent* 2003; 24:589-595.

In: A Window on Surgery and Orthodontics
Editor: Giuseppe Alessandro Scardina ISBN: 978-1-62808-948-6

Chapter IX

Surgical Removal of Genial Tubercles

***Vitor Hugo Leite de Oliveira Rodrigues*[1], *Bruno Gomes Duarte*[1], *Daniel Gomes Salgueiro*[1], *Gabriel Fiorelli Bernini*[2], *Osny Ferreira Júnior*[*3] *and Eduardo Sant' Ana*[3]**

[1]Professionalizing Practice in Oral Surgery, Bauru College of Dentistry, University of São Paulo (FOB-USP), Bauru, São Paulo, Brazil
[2]Stomatology, FOB-USP, Bauru, São Paulo, Brazil
[3]Surgery of the Department of Stomatology and Oral Surgery, FOB-USP, Bauru, São Paulo, Brazil

Abstract

Genial tubercles are tiny bone projections located bilaterally around the lingual foramen, on the lingual face of the mandible.

Purpose: This study intends to present diagnosis methods and surgical techniques to treat this relatively uncommon problem.

Patient: A totally edentulous, 69 year old, female patient came to our clinic complaining of an increase in volume in the floor of the mouth, in the region of the lower central incisors, that was causing instability in the lower total prosthesis.

Results: The surgical planning was the removal of genial tubercle, one week after the surgery no one complication was observed. *Conclusion:* Surgical removal of genial tubercles are a rare situation however in this case this surgery was necessary and no complications was observed after the surgery.

Keywords: Oral surgery, genial tubercles, hypertrophy mandible

[*] Correspondence author: Osny Ferreira Júnior, Departamento de Estomatologia, Disciplina de Cirurgia, Al. Dr. Octávio Pinheiro Brisola, 9-75 - Bauru - SP - Brasil – CEP: 17012-901. Telefone: +55 (14) 32358258. E-mail: osnyfjr@usp.br.

Introduction

Genial tubercles are bone projections located bilaterally around the lingual foramen, on the lingual face, between upper and lower edges of the mandible [1, 2]. The geniohyoid and genioglossus muscles are located there [1-4]. In some cases, these insertions, or the presence of pronounced tubercles, can hinder or impede the use of prosthetic devices [4].

In literature, it is possible to find some complications related to the presence of genial tubercles, such as the fracturing of these structures [2, 5]. This is generally observed in female patients over the age of 67 [2]. Genial tubercle atrophy is also common, especially in atrophic mandibles [1, 2]. Another complication occurs when edentulous patients present resorption of the alveolar process, because then the genial tubercles become pronounced and interfere in prosthesis use. Hypertrophy of these structures affects approximately 1. 45% (+/- 0. 5%) of female patients [3].

Clinical Case

A 69 year old, female patient came to the FOB-USP surgery clinic complaining of an increase in volume in the floor of the mouth, in the region of the lower central incisors, that was causing instability in the lower total prosthesis. During the intraoral clinical exam, it was observed that the patient was totally edentulous and there was ulceration on the floor of the mouth due to trauma from total prosthesis use (Figure 1). Standard lateral teleradiography was performed as well as volume CT-scan (figure 2, 3) to assess local bone structure.

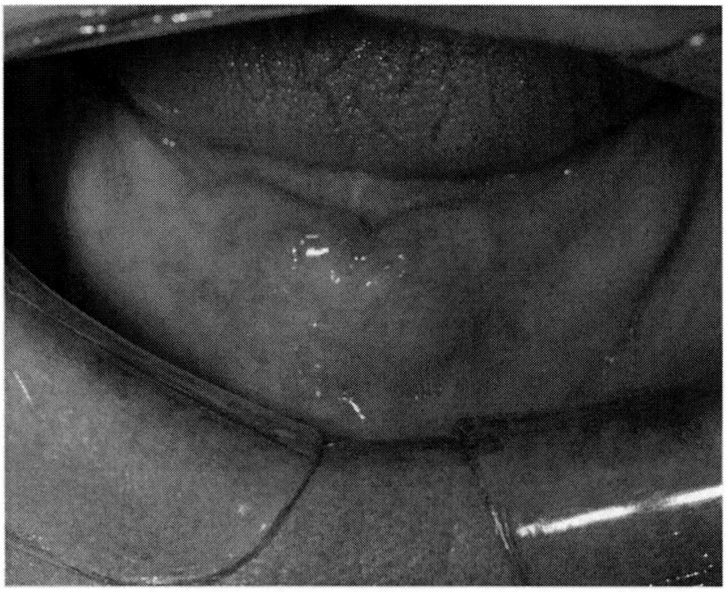

Figure 1. Pre-operative intrabuccal clinical aspect showing the mucosa lesion in the genial tubercle region.

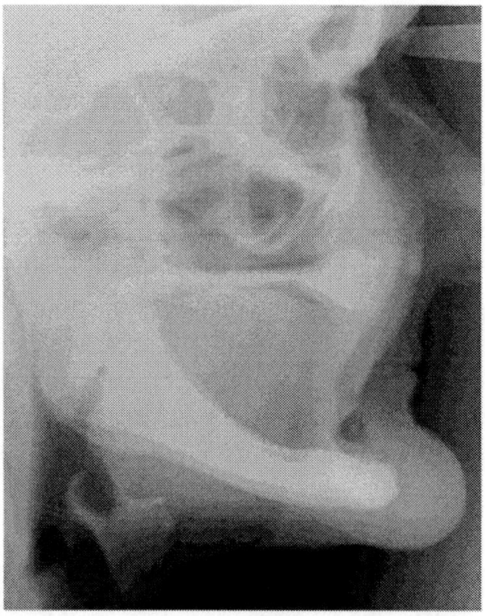

Figure 2. Standard lateral teleradiograph showing the prominence of genial tubercles.

The diagnostic hypothesis was trauma due to genial tubercle protuberance, and this diagnosis was confirmed with the aid of imaging exams. Due to the discomfort caused by these structures to the patient, and the fact the patient does not want to undergo surgery to install osseo-integration implants, the proposed treatment plan was to surgically remove the genial tubercles. Surgery was performed in an outpatient environment under local infiltration and terminal anesthesia. The tubercle region was approached with the help of an incision on the crest of the ridge extending from the pre-molars on one side to the pre-molars on the opposite side, and another incision on the floor of the mouth, parallel to the median sagittal plane. The mucosa was then shifted and the muscles disinserted. Then, the base of the genial tubercles was sectioned using a no. 6 spherical bit.

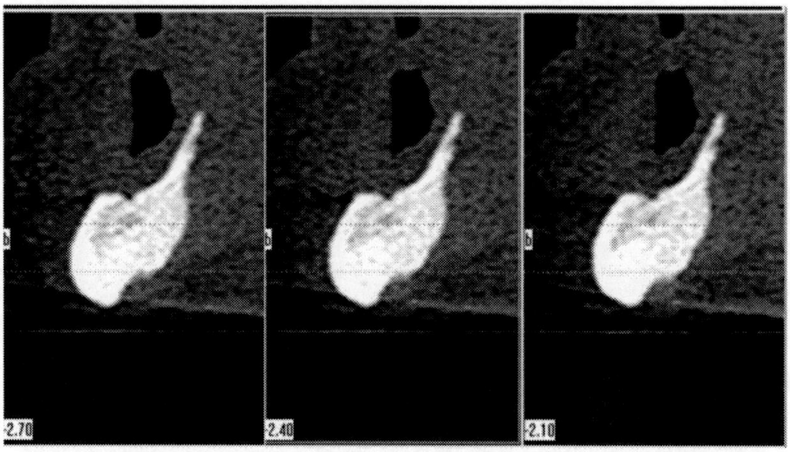

Figure 3. Sagittal cut of the Genial Tubercle region obtained from Cone Beam Volume CT scans (i-Cat).

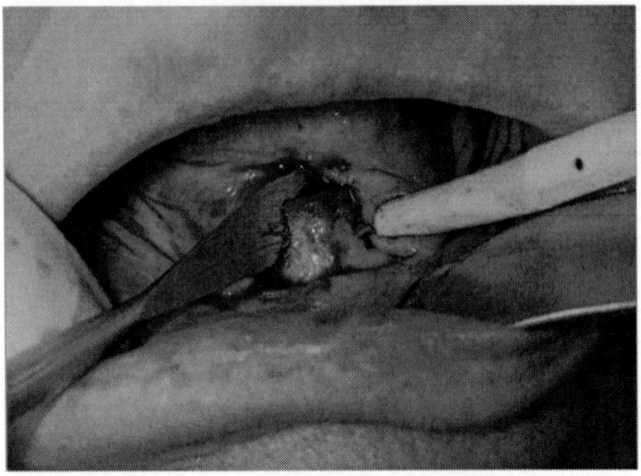

Figure 4. Exposure of genial tubercles.

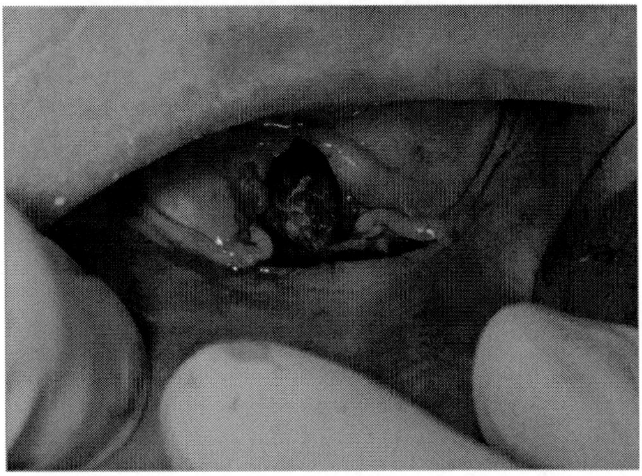

Figure 5. Disinsertion of muscles.

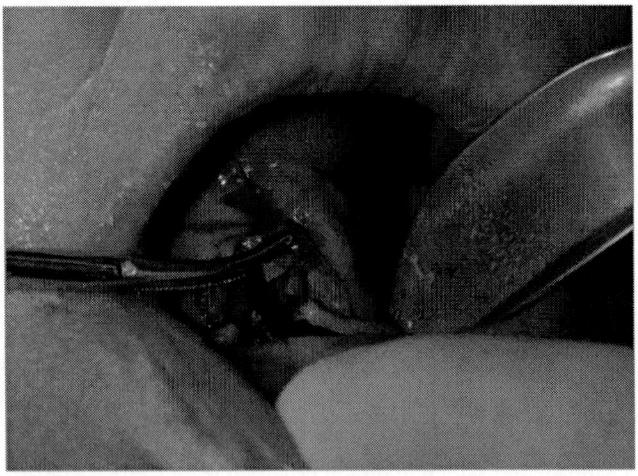

Figure 6. Removal of genial tubercles.

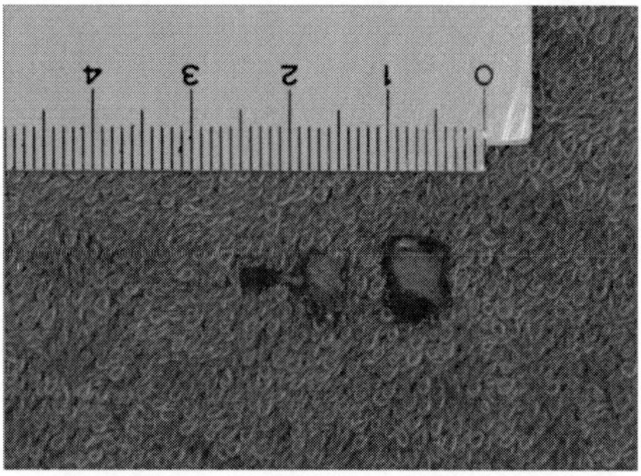

Figure 7. View of removed fragments.

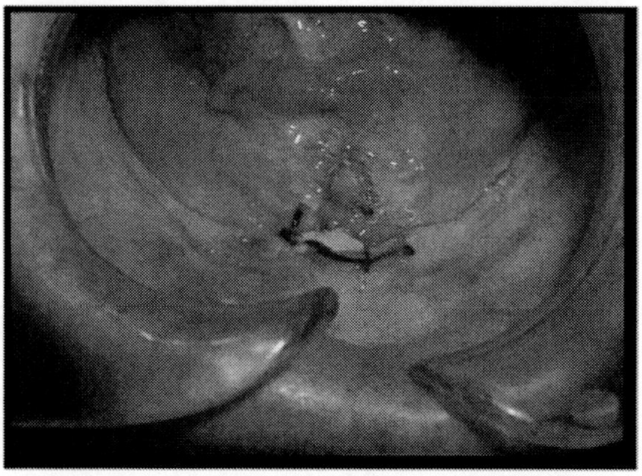

Figure 8. 7 days post-operative.

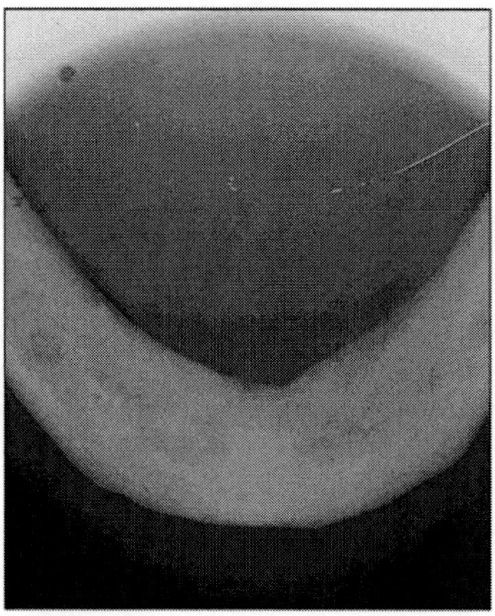

Figure 9. Occlusal radiograph of the mandible during 7-day postoperative control.

The remaining bone fragment was removed and the remaining bone was adjusted using a bone file. The region was sutured using 3-0 silk thread, with simple, interrupted stitches (figures 4-5-6-7).

The stitches were removed one week after the surgical procedure. No clinical alterations were observed at this moment. At the 7-day control, the patient presented good clinical evolution (figure 8). An occlusal radiograph was taken (figure 9) and the patient was forwarded to have new prostheses made.

Discussion

Genial tubercles usually are small bony protuberances on the lingual aspect of the mandible symphysis [6], according to Greyling [3], no important function can be attributed to the presence and size of genial tubercles. However, some authors comment on the importance of the structure's correct location in mandibular advancement surgeries, in patients with obstructive sleep apnea syndrome (SAAS) [7]. A study conducted by Hueman [7] with the objective of assessing the correct location of upper and lower genial tubercles, used volume CT scans (cone beam).

According to the author, use of the cone beam CT scan is valid for assessing the location of these structures because due to their location, the assessment of tubercles using panoramic or occlusal radiographs may be jeopardized. Thus, the main objective of using CT scans is to allow better visualization of these structures and more accurate measures (without distortions).

According to the literature we can increase8 or enlargement [6,9] of the genial tubercles, a fact that may be responsible to painful symptoms or poorly adapt of the prosthesis. In this work the painful symptoms and poor adaptation of prosthesis is related mandibular atrophy and a more superficial position of these structures. Similar cases can be found in the literature, where the enlargement of the genital tubercles and mandibular bone resorption were responsible for poorly adaptation of the prosthesis and painful swelling [6]. In this is the surgical removal of the genial tubercles is the treatment of this case. Another important aspect to underscore is what happens with the muscles that insert themselves in the genial tubercles after their removal. According to Petterson [4], reinsertion of the genioglossus muscle occurs randomly, and according to Maw [10], there are 3 different explanations for the tongue's protrusion movement after disinsertion of the genioglossus muscle: The intrinsic muscles can adjust in such a way that projects the tongue slightly forward. The palatoglossus muscle, acting isolatedly, can lift the tongue and move it anteriorly.

After the fracture of the genial tubercle, the remaining fibers of the genioglossus muscle can maintain the tongue's capacity to protrude. The surgical technique used to remove genial tubercles also aims at reinserting the geniohyoid and genioglossus muscles. The technique described in this case is simple to apply, has excellent postoperative results and the complete oral rehabilitation of the patients.

Finally, it is worth underscoring that removal is opted for when the patient is not submitted to grafts to increase the alveolar edge. In that case, it is suggested to keep the genial tubercles because they help in the region's bone reconstruction.

References

[1] Gallego L, Junquera L, Villarreal P, Vicente JC. Spontaneous fracture of the mandibular genial tubercles. A case report. *Med. Oral Patol Oral Cir. Bucal* 2007; 12: E599-601.

[2] Shohat I, Shoshani Y, Taicher S. Fracture of the genial tubercles associated with a mandibular denture: A clinical report. *J. Prosthet Dent* 2003; 89: 232-33.

[3] Greyling LM, Le Grange F, Meiring JH. Mandibular Spine: A Case Report. *Clinical Anatomy* 1997; 10: 416-8.

[4] Spagnoli DB, Gollehon SG, Misiek DJ (2008) Cirurgia Pré-Protética. In: Princípios de Cirurgia BucoMaxiloFacial 2008, Vol 1, Miloro M, Ghali GE, Larsen P, Waite PD Eds, Editora Santos, São Paulo, 158-187.

[5] Yaedú RYF, Rubira-Bullen IRF, Sant'Ana E. Spontaneous fracture of genial tubercles: case report. *Quintessence Int.* 2006; 37: 737-9.

[6] Rubira-Bullen IRF, Sant'Ana E, Yaedú RYF, Tolentino ES, Borgo E. Rare enlargement of the genial tubercles. *Surgical and Radiologic Anatomy.* [Epub Ahead of print].

[7] Hueman EM, Noujeim ME, Langlais RP, Prihoda TJ, Miller FR: Accuracy of cone beam computed tomography in determining the location of the genial tubercle. *Otolaryngology–Head and Neck Surgery* 2007; 137: 115-58.

[8] Wiesenbaugh JM, Bingham C. Sialolithiasis and enlarged genial tubercles. *Oral Surg Oral Med. Oral Pathol* 1970; 30: 506-7.

[9] Greyling LM, Le Grange F, Meiring JH. Mandibular Spine: a case report. *Clin Anat* 1997; 10: 416-8.

[10] Maw Rb, Lindsay JS. Conservative management of genial tubercle fracture. *Oral Surg Oral Med Oral Pathol.* 1970; 30: 445-9.

In: A Window on Surgery and Orthodontics
Editor: Giuseppe Alessandro Scardina
ISBN: 978-1-62808-948-6

Chapter X

Hinge Axis - An Overview

Ashu Sharma*, G. R. Rahul†, Soorya T. Poduval‡, and Karunakar Shetty#
[1]Department of Prosthodontics,
Bangalore Institute of Dental Sciences and Research Center,
Wilson Garden, Bangalore, India

Abstract

Transverse hinge axis is defined as, an imaginary line around which the mandible may rotate within the sagittal plane. Mandibular movements around this horizontal axis is an opening and closing motion and are referred to as a hinge movement. The hinge movement is probably the only example of mandibular activity in which pure rotational movement occurs. A lot of discussion has taken place in past over mandibular hinge axis. The dental profession recognizes the importance of hinge axis. A thorough understanding of various concepts involved in hinge axis is of prime importance. The purpose of this article is to give a complete overview about everything that one needs to know about hinge axis including different types and methods of locating hinge axis and its clinical application in prosthodontic treatment.

A PubMed search of English literature was conducted up to January 2010 using the terms related to hing axis. Additionally, the bibliographies of 5 previous reviews, their cross references as well as articles published in dental journals were manually searched.

Keywords: Hinge axis, Transverse hinge axis, Terminal hinge axis, Mandibular hinge axis, Kinematic hinge axis

Transverse hinge axis is defined as, an imaginary line around which the mandible may rotate within the sagittal plane. [1] Mandibular movements around this horizontal axis is an

* Email: drashu_sharma@yahoo.com.
† Email: rahulaparna@hotmail.com.
‡ Email: soorypodu@hotmail.com.
# Email: dr_karu@yahoo.com.

opening and closing motion and are referred to as a hinge movement. The hinge movement is probably the only example of mandibular activity in which pure rotational movement occurs. When the condyles are in their most superior position in the articular fossae and the mouth is purely rotated open, the axis around which movement occurs is called terminal hinge axis. In centric relation the mandible can be rotated around the horizontal axis to a distance of only 20 to 25mm, as measured between the incisal edges of the maxillary and mandibular incisors. [2]

Search Strategy

A PubMed search of English literature was conducted up to January 2010 using the terms: Hinge axis, Transverse hinge axis, Terminal hinge axis, Mandibular hinge axis, Kinematic hinge axis. Additionally, the bibliographies of 5 previous reviews, their cross references as well as articles published in Journal of American Dental Association, Journal of Oral Rehabilitation, British Dental Journal, Journal of Prosthetic Dentistry and Journal of Collegium Antropologicum were manually searched.

History and Review of Literature [3]

Campion [4, 5], produced probably the first graphic record of mandibular movements on a patient. He used a basic form of pantograph which produced a succession of dots on the skin of the side of the face as the condyles moved during function. Bennett [6], in his classical paper on movements of the mandible, stated that no single fixed centre of rotation for the mandible existed since the centre of rotation constantly shifted (for movements in the sagittal plane). However, he did point out that the mandible was capable of two independent movements; one, an angular rotation about the condyle, the other a translation movement produced by the gliding of the condyle along its path.

In 1939 McCollum [7, 8, 9] published a very important series of articles concerning restorative remedies. He was one of the leading advocates of the 'hinge-axis theory'. McCollum described how he came to demonstrate conclusively the existence of a definite opening and closing axis by using a face-bow rigidly attached to the lower teeth with orthodontic appliances. The development of accurate and rigid clutches, and adjustable face-bows, led to the determination of the hinge-axis easily. He also demonstrated, by means of diagrams showing exact locations of nine pairs of hinge-axis points and that external landmarks were of little use in location of the axis.

In 1955 Collett [10] stated: 'There is not agreement on the existence of the hinge-axis. It is important to those who believe in its existence, because by using it we can record centric relation at a level above the place where the proprioceptive reflex occurs, transfer our recording to an articulating instrument, and on the instrument, close down to the occlusal level'.

Kornfield [11] discussed the anatomy of the temporomandibular joints and outlined the technique of recording the hinge-axis and its transfer to the articulator. He stated that the location of the hinge-axis was the basis of all articulator transfers, and made the study and treatment of masticatory disease easier and more intelligible. Schallhorn [12] discussed the advantages and disadvantages of an arbitrary hinge-axis location for face-bow transfer compared with a kinematic location. Page [13] stated that there were at least twelve hinge axes in every head; three in each temporomandibular joint and three in each mandibular angle. These, he said, were responsible for movements in all three planes.

Weinberg [14] attempted to clear up any misunderstanding concerning the hinge-axis in the following way. He pointed out it was essential to use the terminal or 'trained' mandibular hinge movement. Although criticism had been leveled at the recording of the trained hinge movement because patients usually functioned with condylar translation, he pointed out that this recording was the static starting point for functional mandibular movements. On the subject of transographics, or the two transverse hinge axes theory, Weinberg [14] pointed out that much of the concept was based on the asymmetry of the condyles. However, he pointed out that 'off-centre' opening and closing movements of the mandible were still perpendicular to the transverse hinge-axis. He said that movement in one direction in the plane could have only one axis of rotation and that two axial centers of rotation for the same plane and movement was a self-contradictory statement.

Lauritzen and Bodner [15] used fifty patients to determine variations in hinge-axis location when compared with arbitrary methods. It was found that their method of hinge-axis location gave 67% of the points at a distance of 5-13 mm from the arbitrary points. When the arbitrary centre was changed to an area of 5 mm radius, only 76% of the hinge-axis locations were within this. In view of the differences in opinion, Trapozzano and Lazzari [16] in 1961 decided to re-examine two problems (i) Whether there was a terminal hinge-axis, and (ii) if there was, whether or not only one existed. The investigators located what they thought to be the terminal hinge-axis in fourteen subjects, but left the final decision to a group of neutral observers. They found that 57 2% of the subjects had more than one condyle hinge-axis point on either one or both sides and concluded that the high degree of infallibility attributed to hinge-axis points should be seriously questioned. It is interesting that this conclusion differed somewhat from early statements.

Aull[17] published a paper in which he described four main schools of thought regarding the hinge-axis: (1) the absolute location of the hinge-axis school, as practiced by Lucia (1953), McCollum (1939, 1943), Granger (1952, 1954) etc. (2) the arbitrary axis school as practiced by Craddock & Symmons (1952). (3) the non-believers, such as Beck (1959), who thought the axis to be theoretically possible but not practically acceptable; (4) the split hinge-axis school who believed in the transographic theory, such as Slavens (1961). Aull performed experiments to show the relative accuracy of the method used to locate the terminal hinge position and demonstrated the fallacy of the split axis theory. In 1970, Long [18] described an intra-oral technique for locating the terminal hinge-axis by using two accurate centric relation records at two different degrees of jaw separation.

In 1995, in a study [19] with the subtraction technique, 15 TMJs were radiographically investigated in RP for change of condylar position in relation to the glenoid fossa after insertion of an anterior bite plane that caused an increase of the vertical dimension of 4 to 7 mm. All condyles changed position (range 0. 31 to 1. 84 mm), which indicates that pure rotation did not occur. The direction of condylar movement varied not only among subjects but also between the two condyles of each subject. One clinical implication of this study may be that increasing vertical dimension in prosthodontic rehabilitation should be done with caution in regard to the reliability of the recorded transverse horizontal axis. In addition, an increase of the occlusal vertical dimension does not necessarily mean an increase of the joint space. Instead, it may become narrower.

An investigating study [20] was done with the aim to determine the spatial relations of the Terminal hinge axis of the Temporomandibular joints toward arbitrary point proposed by Sumiya Hobo (H) and Frankfurt horizontal (FH). The sample consisted of 50 examinees. Terminal hinge axis was located, using Lauritzen's technique, on the left side of face for each examinee. Arbitrary point, as proposed by Sumiya Hobo, was measured and point Orbital was defined by palpation. On designated points steel pellets 0. 25 mm in diameter were stocked. Lathero--latheral cephalogram was obtained for each examinee. Cephalograms were traced down on a transparent foil and points Orbital, THA--terminal hinge axis, Hobo and Porion--as the uppermost point of the metal ear rod of the cephalostat, were designated. Connecting points Orbital and Porion, Frankfurt horizontal was defined, and shortest distance toward points THA and Hobo, as well as between them were measured. Lines parallel and perpendicular to Frankfurt horizontal were drawn through point THA. In a co-ordinate system defined in such a way, upper left quadrant was first, upper right second, lower right third, and lower left was fourth. Observation was made in which quadrant Hobo point was located. Measured values were statistically evaluated. Results revealed that Hobo point is located in first quadrant in 5 cases, in second in 7, third quadrant in 18, and in fourth in 20 cases. That means that Hobo point is located lower to the THA point in majority of our population. Points THA and Hobo were not identical in any case. Mean values of variables showed that investigated points were inferior to the FH. Measures of variability revealed great variability of both points toward FH, as well as for their mutual distance. It could be pointed out that THA point should be defined kinematically during prosthodontic procedures, and that orientation in articulator's space should not be according to the FH.

In 2001, Bowley et al. [21] investigated the magnitude and types of occlusal errors produced by deviations between the patient’s transverse horizontal axis and the axle on the articulator. A simplified monoplane model was diagrammatically analyzed for deviations from the model’s true transverse horizontal axis. Axis deviations of 5 mm were used in 8 different directions from the true transverse horizontal axis of the model. Changes in the orientation of the mandibular plane to the maxillary plane were illustrated diagrammatically. These changes were quantified by geometric and trigonometric assessments. The results showed that all axis deviations produced mandibular plane orientation errors with angular plane malalignment to the maxillary plane on complete closure. These axis deviations also produced anterior-posterior shifting of the mandibular plane relative to the maxillary plane.

In 2002 an in vivo study [22] was done which compared the location of an anatomically predetermined hinge axis point with the determined kinematic axis. Forty subjects (27 males, 13 females; 23 to 47 years of age) with functionally acceptable occlusion and no detectable clinical signs of temporomandibular disorders participated in the study. The earpiece alignment flags on a mechanical SAM Axiograph III combination flag/face-bow were used to locate the right and left predetermined hinge axis points, 10 mm anterior to the earpiece. The right and left kinematic center of rotation was located as described by Lauritzen and confirmed with the PC Axiotron electronic Axiograph to within 0. 25 mm. the results suggest that the predetermined axis point is well within the clinical norm for estimated location of the transverse horizontal mandibular axis.

In 2004, Preston [23] discussed the history and development of the hinge-axis concept, particularly in relation to colinear and non-colinear theories.

There are few other studies which are somehow related to locating mandibular hinge axis. A study done by Thieme KM et al. [24] tried to evaluate the mandibularly fixed hinge axis (MFHA) for patients who had problems with their temporo-mandibular joints. They thought that the results could also provide information on the reason for the distortion of the movement of the TMJs, which cannot be yielded by X-ray radiographs.

Konate NY et al. [25] did a study related to hinge axis. The objective of this work was to determinate the average value of the condylar slope of Black African subject and to set up its variation according to whether the localization of the hinge axis is real or arbitrary. The results of this study revealed that the average value of the slope condylar is 44,28 degrees in arbitrary hinge axis and 45,7 degrees in hinge axis real; and this difference is not statistically significant.

In 2010 Tokiwa H et al. [26] conducted a study to determine anatomical locations of the hinge axis point, kinematic axis point and reference point for the palpated lateral condylar pole on lateral cephalograms. Subjects comprised 18 Japanese women selected according to following criteria: normal occlusion; and absence of signs and symptoms of stomatognathic function. Lateral cephalograms were used to determine anatomical locations of the three points in the condyle. Mean location of hinge axis point was 12. 9 mm anterior of the porion and 5. 3 mm inferior to the Frankfort horizontal plane, the kinematic axis point was situated in 12. 8 mm anterior and 0. 1 mm inferior, and the reference point for the palpated lateral condylar pole was situated 10. 7 mm anterior and 0. 8 mm inferior, respectively. The kinematic axis point was located outside the condyle in the majority of subjects.

Different Theories of Transverse Hinge Axis [17]

From the early experiments four main schools of thought have evolved regarding the horizontal axis. They are as follows:

Group 1:- Absolute Location theory of Transverse Axis

There are those [27] who believe that there is a definite transverse axis and it should be located as accurately as possible. I feel that the investigators who endorse this concept have established a repeatable point of orientation from which the following information and relationships may be obtained:

1. With the aid of the face-bow, it is possible to relate the maxillary cast to the transverse axis of the articulator in the same relationship as the maxillae are related to the anatomic mandibular axis through the condyles.
2. The mandibular hinge axis is coincided with and related to the maxillary hinge axis by means of a centric relation record.
3. The path of closure on the terminal hinge will, therefore, be the same on the articulator as in the mouth.

Group 2:- Arbitrary Theory of Transverse Axis Location

The second group includes those who believe that an accurate location of the terminal hinge position would be of some value, but do not believe that it has enough value over an arbitrary location to be worth the added effort necessary to locate it. Craddock[28] states, "But the search for the axis, in addition to being troublesome, is of no more than academic interest, for it will never be found to lie more than a few millimeters distant from the assumed center in the condyle itself. As is well known, this may be determined by simple palpation or by following the convention of measuring a distance of about 1 cm anteriorly along a line drawn from the upper free margin of the tragus of the ear to the corner of the eye."

Their argument is sound as far as it goes. However, according to the thinking of Group-1, Group-2 fails to recognize that if the hinge axis of the articulator does not coincide with the hinge axis of the patient, the path of closure will not be the same.

Group 3:- Non Believers Theory of Transverse Axis Location

Then, there is a third group who believe it is impossible to locate the terminal hinge position with accuracy. There are many of this group who believe the transverse axis is theoretical, but not practical. The word "accuracy" must be reduced to terms of degree. As an example, if the dentist could locate the terminal hinge position consistently within a radius of 1 mm, this certainly would be more acceptable than a location with a variance of a 2 mm. radius. Actually, neither one is accurate, but the first is certainly more accurate than the second. It is understandable that the sense of perception and delicacy of touch are keener in some individuals than others. Lauritzen and Wolford[29] confirm this, and Kurth and Feinstein [30] using an articulator and a working model to locate the hinge axis, found any number of points within a range of 2 mm. that could be considered a point of rotation or non-movement. The opening and closing movement was limited to approximately 10 to 11 degrees. Borgh and Posselts could not record the axis on a modified Hanau H articulator without errors. The errors amounted to 1 to 1. 5 mm. at a 10 to 15 degree opening.

Group 4:- Split-Axis Rotation Theory

Group 4 includes those who follow the Transograph theory. Followers of this theory believe in the "split-axis" with which each condyle rotates independently of the other. Inasmuch as the mandible is not bilaterally symmetrical, and the terminal hinge position mark on one side of the face is usually a little higher than it is on the other side of the face (relative to their respective landmarks), it would follow that there cannot be a common axis. There must be two axes parallel to each other with both axes at right angles to the opening and closing movements of the mandible.

Arthur E. Aull performed an experiment to show a method to locate the terminal hinge axis and also to demonstrate the fallacy of the split-axis theory.

Methods of Locating Hinge Axis

Different methods have been used to locate and transfer the hinge axis to the articulator which can be divided into three groups- arbitrary group, kinematic group and modified techniques. . These are briefly discussed below.

I. Arbitrary methods
II. Kinematic methods

III. Modified techniques
A. Loma-linda hinge axis recording device and method.
B. Buhnergraph intraoral method.
C. Technique using geometric principle to locate hinge axis.
D. Abdal-Hadi's technique of locating arbitrary hinge axis.

I. Arbitrary Methods of Hinge Axis Location

Many dentists use arbitrary posterior reference points based on average, anatomic landmarks considered reasonably accurate for most clinical situations. Arbitrary axis points determined from anatomical landmarks are popular due to their ease of the use compared to trial-and-error method of locating the kinematic axis. It has been demonstrated mathematically that location of an arbitrary axis point ± 5 mm anterior-posterior to the kinematic axis will result in negligible error (0. 2 mm) on the nonworking side when a 3-mm–thick centric relation record is used. [22]

1. 1 cm in front of the line from the apex of the tragus of the ear to the outer canthus of the eye, given by Fenn et al. in 1961. [31]
2. 11 to 13 mm anterior to the upper one-third of the tragus of the ear on a line extending to the outer canthus of the eye, given by Henderson et al. in 1973. [32]
3. 13 mm anterior to the posterior margin of the center of the tragus of the ear on a line extending to the corner of the eye, given by Osborne et al. in 1968. [33]
4. 10 mm anterior to the center of a spherical insert for the external auditory meatus and 7 mm below the Frankfort horizontal plane. [34]
5. Palpation. This method was applied as described by Dawson. [35] From a position behind the patient, the index finger was placed over the joint area, and the patient was asked to open widely. As the condyle translated forward, the fingertip was dropped into the depression left by the protruded condyle.
6. The Gysi point located 13 mm in front of the most upper part of the external auditory meatus on a line passing to the ectocanthion. [36]
7. The Lejoyeux point situated 10 to II mm in front of the ear on a line to the canthus and 5 mm below it. [37]
8. The Lauritzen- Bodner axis determined by the use of specially constructed disks 10 mm in diameter and a plastic ruler. This point is located 12 mm anterior and 2 mm below the porion. [15]

While it is desirable to place an arbitrary axis as close as possible to the kinematic one, the results obtained indicate that none of the arbitrary methods used was ideal for locating the hinge axis. In a study done by Mohmoud K. A. Razek, [38] in which five methods were used to locate the arbitrary hinge axis of the mandible on 120 dentulous patients. The obtained axes were compared with the kinematic axis which had been located on each patient. While none of the arbitrary methods used proved to be ideal for locating the hinge axis, the axis located by Dawson's palpation method fell consistently closer to the kinematic axis. A combination of the arbitrary methods should therefore be used if it is not feasible to record the axis kinematically [38].

II. Kinematic Method

The kinematic axis was recorded for each patient using a Hanau Kinematic Transfer Bow. Differet authors have used different methods. The consensus is that a hinge axis locator and kinematic face-bow provide the most accurate method of mounting. [39]

As explained in a study by Palik et al., [39] the kinematic face-bow uses the terminal hinge axis and inferior orbital rim as reference points. The area of the true hinge axis was located by palpating the subject's condyles during opening and closing of the mandible. A hinge axis flagging device (TMJ Instrument Co. , Inc. , Santa Ana, Calif.), worn like a pair of glasses and secured posteriorly by a head strap, was adjusted to the subject. The subject was then positioned at approximately a 45- to 60-degree angle from horizontal.

After a clutch tray was rigidly affixed to the mandibular teeth with Impregum (Premier Dental Products Co., Norristown, Pa.), the Hanau No. 135-6 kinematic face-bow (Teledyne Dental Co., Hanau Division, Buffalo, N. Y.) was firmly attached to the clutch stem. The condylar pointers were provisionally positioned, and the subject was instructed to open and close within a limited range of approximately 1 cm. During these movements, the subject was maintained in centric relation with light but continuous hand pressure. The condylar pointers were adjusted until they were directly perpendicular to the hinge axis and rotated without translatory movement.

With the mandible maintained in centric relation, the axis points were tattooed on the skin and the hinge axis locating equipment was removed. A bite fork (Teledyne Dental Co.) was adapted to the occlusal surfaces of the maxillary teeth with black modeling compound in cake form (Kerr/Sybron Mfg. Co., Romulus, Mich.) in each subject. The modeling compound was cooled and trimmed to leave only a light index of the cusp tips. The maxillary cast was positioned in the modeling compound index to ensure accuracy of fit. The bite fork was used for both kinematic and arbitrary face-bow recordings.

The bite fork was placed in the mouth and the kinematic face-bow firmly attached. The condylar pointers were adjusted to the terminal hinge axis points with the patient in the same postural position. The orbital pointer was positioned at the inferior orbital foramen, previously identified by palpation. The kinematic facebow was then carefully transferred to the Hanau No. 158-3 arcon articulator (Teledyne Dental Co.). The face-bow was positioned to relate each condylar pointer accurately to the corresponding apparatus on the articulator. The orbital pointer was positioned by adjusting the cast-supporting device attached to the base of the articulator. The maxillary cast was seated and secured in the compound index and mounted to the articulator.

Modified Plexiglas (Rohm and Haas, Philadelphia, Pa.) disks were positioned on the lateral aspect of each condylar element of the articulator parallel to the sagittal plane. The disks had perpendicular, horizontal, and vertical lines etched on their outer surfaces, and the lines intersected at the exact point of the terminal hinge axis on the articulator. On each Plexiglas disk, a self-adhesive TMJ graph circle (TMJ Instrument Co., Inc.) was placed with its 0 coordinate point coinciding with the horizontal and vertical line intersection to simulate an x-y graph. The subject's identification, side of articulator (right or left), and anteroposterior positions were identified on the graph circles.

III. Modified Techniques

This group includes techniques used to locate arbitrary and kinematic hinge axis by making some modifications in conventional methods.

A. Loma-linda Hinge Axis Recording Device and Method [40]

The opponents of use of a kinematic hinge-axis location for edentulous patients point to its unreliability because of the resiliency of the oral mucosa, the added weight of the recording clutch which tends to shift the denture base, and the time-consuming nature of the procedure. To eliminate some of these disadvantages, we have developed a modification of the Loma Linda hinge-axis recording device and face-bows for use on edentulous patients.

Modification of the Hinge-Axis Locator

1. Cut two parallel channels down the length of a clear Lucite plastic blank to accommodate the hinge-axis recorder and flags.
2. Modify a set of lower edentulous impression trays with cold-curing acrylic resin to accommodate the modified Lucite blank.
3. Cut a pair of hollow tubes, four in all, 1/2 inch in length.
4. Perforate each of the aluminum trays, and shorten the handle.
5. Fix the Lucite blank and hollow tubes to the trays with a mix of cold-curing acrylic resin. The resin is allowed to harden, chemically locking the Lucite to the tray as a new handle and mechanically locking the tubes as stabilizers for a circum-mandibular elastic effect. The acrylic resin covers all external portions of the edentulous trays and is smoothed and contoured to eliminate all sharp and rough edges. A series of lower impression trays can thus be modified to make clutches for use with the Loma Linda hinge-axis locator.

B. Buhnergraph Intraoral Method [18]

It is the technique used to record terminal hinge axis, with the help of an instrument which can be made by the dentist called Buhnergraph. It is named after Dr. W. A. Buhner of Daytona Beach, Florida, who has helped with its design and machine work.

In the article by James Hart Long, an intraoral technique for locating the terminal hinge axis has been described. The key to the success of this technique lies in the accurate location of centric relation at 2 different degrees of jaw separation. Centric relation can be located by many techniques but there is some variability in the results obtained by any of them. Therefore, each dentist should have a means of comparing his registrations so that an intelligent selection can be made. The Buhnergraph and the technique described here provide a means of locating centric relation and determining and/or verifying the location of the terminal hinge axis.

Buhnergraph instrument consists of a U-shaped piece of aluminum which is attached to the underside of the lower member of a Whip Mix articulator. On each side is attached an adjustable arm containing a pointed shaft which moves in and out.

Casts are mounted on the articulator with the maxillary cast preferably related to the terminal hinge axis and the mandibular cast related to the maxillary cast by means of a tentative centric relation record. The pointed shafts are adjusted to fit into the recess on each lateral face of the condylar guide housing. These recesses mark the center of rotation of the articulator. A piece of graph paper is now fastened to the lateral face of each condylar guide housing and the horizontal graph lines are made parallel to the upper member of the articulator. With the removal of the condylar elements, the instrument ceases to be an articulator and becomes a Buhnergraph. The tentative centric relation registration record is placed between the casts and the relationship is carefully stabilized.

C. Technique Using Geometric Principle to Locate Hinge Axis [41]

Gunderson and Parker presented a technique that uses geometric principles to locate the mandibular transverse horizontal axis (hinge axis). This technique is a rapid method for locating the mandibular transverse horizontal axis of a patient with accuracy. It does not use an arbitrary posterior reference point, which introduces unnecessary errors where maximum precision is indicated. In addition it is a technique useful in teaching the concept of hinge rotation to the student of mandibular movement.

1. A millimeter graph paper is attached to the facial sidearm of a hinge axis locator (TMJ Instrument Co., Santa Ana, Calif.) positioned over the site of the temporomandibular joint.
2. A clutch is rigidly attached to the mandibular teeth and a microadjustable axis location assembly (TM J Instrument Co.) is placed over the millimeter grid.
3. A graphic stylus is inserted in place of the axis locator pin and positioned in the anterior region of the graph paper.
4. A series of arcs are scribed by gently guiding the patient in repeated retruded (hinge) opening movements and adjusting the mandibular sidearm to position the stylus in a series of positions located on the grid.
5. The procedure is repeated in an area of the grid inferior to the temporomandibular joint.
6. One or more of the arcs are selected from the anterior and inferior groupings. A line is scribed perpendicular to a tangent of each of these arcs (or center of the chord of each arc). The point where these lines intersect is the center of rotation, or the hinge axis reference point (Fig 3).
7. An alternative technique is to identify a horizontal and vertical grid line that is perpendicular to a scribed arc from the anterior and inferior groups. The intersection of these grid lines also identifies the center of rotation and quickly locates a reference point for the mandibular transverse horizontal axis.
8. Once the intersecting point has been located, the graphic stylus is replaced with an axis locator pin. The locator pin is positioned precisely over the marked grid point and locked in place. The hinge axis may be verified with conventional arcing techniques.
9. The grid is removed and the hinge axis point is transferred to the patient as a posterior reference point for subsequent procedures.
10. The procedure is repeated on the opposite side. Two reference points, once located, provide an accurate determination of the mandibular transverse horizontal axis.

D. Abdal-Hadi's Technique of Locating Arbitrary Hinge Axis [36]

Abdal-Hadi proposed a new arbitrary method. The author's point is based on the high correlation between the width profile of the face and the X coordinate of the kinematic point. Thus the use of the linear regression formula permits prediction of the anterioposterior site of the kinematic point. This equation is Y = 9. 5 c 0. 95 (X) where Y represents the width profile of the face measured from the ectocanthion to the center of the external auditory meatus and X is equal to the anterioposterior position of the kinematic point. A constant distance equal to 0.5 mm was used above the line passing from the center of the external auditory meatus to the canthus to locate the superioinferior position of the proposed method.

The proposed arbitrary method of recording the hinge axis based on the correlation between the profile width of the face and the kinematic axis was compared with three commonly used arbitrary methods. Furthermore, this method clearly illustrated that its highest concentration was in the posteriosuperior quarter around the true axis. The proposed technique was found to be more accurate than the other techniques.

Rationale of Hinge Axis

According to Weinberg [14], the transverse hinge axis plus one other anterior point serves to locate the maxillae in space, three separate points, or one hinge axis and an anterior point, are required to orientate any solid object in space. The interocclusal centric relation recordings are made in wax. The location of the transverse hinge axis serves only to orientate the maxillae and to record the static starting point for functional mandibular movements. It does not record centric relation or condylar movements. Intraoral eccentric records are used with the Hanau type of adjustable articulator to estimate the functional condylar movements concerned with cuspal occlusion.

Chair-side and laboratory procedures could be considerably shortened if an accurate hinge axis could be located and transferred to an adjustable articulator for edentulous patients. [40] Once objective is achieved, dentists can [40] (1) Alter the vertical dimension of occlusion on the articulator. [42] (2) Obtain the centric relation records and verify them at the try-in at an altered vertical dimension of occlusion. (3) Minimize the remounting procedures to perfect the occlusal scheme. (4) Safely use a cusp-form (anatomic) posterior tooth where indicated with minimal occlusal adjustments. (5) Develop an occlusion which would preserve and restore oral function.

The anatomic or the kinematic hinge axis face-bow transfer is the first step in recording the relationship of the maxillary arch to the condylar paths. These two methods of maxillary cast orientation differ basically only in accuracy. Once the maxillary cast is oriented on the articulator, the centric relation record completes the static, or starting, relationship between the maxillae and the condyles in the temporomandibular fossae. [43]

Interest in condylar movement dates back to the middle of the nineteenth century. [44] However, Snow's face-bow, proposed in 1899, represents the first instrument designed to transfer the position of the horizontal axis from the patient to the articulator. There has been considerable debate about whether it is clinically useful to locate the axis, and whether an arbitrary point on the face can be satisfactorily substituted for a kinematic axis. [40] Gordon et al. [45] published an article on these two controversial points. The purpose of this investigation was to mathematically calculate the amount of cusp height and mesiodistal error at the second molar that results from incorrect location of the terminal hinge axis of 5 and 8 mm to the anterior, posterior, superior, and inferior. With jaw relation records 3 and 6 mm thick at the incisors, the errors in cusp height at the second molar ranged from 0. 15 mm open space to 0. 4 mm excess height. The mesiodistal error ranged from 0. 51 mm toward the distal to 0. 52 mm toward the mesial. While the mesiodistal component to the error has been calculated in the past with some accuracy, the values obtained have varied because different anatomic dimensions were used. In addition, the vertical component of the error in cusp height was not considered and/or not subjected to in-depth calculation.

Summary and Conclusion

A theoretic discussion of the transverse hinge axis has been presented in relation to some of the controversial concepts. Most arbitrary axis point locations recommended in the literature will create 6 mm or more of error. A minimal error of 5 mm can be expected no matter what arbitrary position might be chosen. Placement of the tragus-canthus line at the superior border of the tragus of the ear will contribute to greater inaccuracy in most patients. The largest percentage of true axis locations will be inferior to the tragus-canthus line at the superior border of the tragus of the ear. [46]

In the final analysis, the true value of our individual work can be measured only by the degree of fineness with which we practice the art of dentistry rather than by the particular school of thought to which we adhere. [14]

References

[1] The glossary of prosthodontic terms. *J Prosthet Dent.* 2005; 94:10-92.

[2] Okesson. J. P. *management of temporomandibular disorders and occlusion.* 5th ed. Missouri-Mosby, 2003.

[3] Winstanley RB. The hinge-axis: a review of the literature. *J Oral Rehabil.* 1985;12:135-59.

[4] Campion GG. A method of recording graphically the movements of the mandibular condyles in the living subject. *British Dental Journal.* 1902; 23: 713.

[5] Campion GG. Some graphic records of movements of the mandible in the living subject and their bearing on the mechanism of the joint and the construction of articulators. *Dental Cosmos.* 1905; 47:39.

[6] Bennett NG. A contribution to the study of the movements of the mandible. *Proceeding of the Royal Society of Medicine.* 1908;1:79.

[7] McCollum BB. Fundamentals involved in prescribing restorative dental remedies. *Part I. Dental Items of Interest.* 1939; 61:522.

[8] McCollum BB. Fundamentals involved in prescribing restorative dental remedies. *Part II. Dental Items of Interest.* 1939; 61:724.

[9] McCollum BB. Fundamentals involved in prescribing restorative dental remedies. *Part III. Dental Items of Interest.* 1939; 61:852.

[10] Collett HA. The movements of the temporomandibular joint and their relation to the problems of occlusion. *J Prosthet Dent.* 1955; 5: 486.

[11] Kornfield M. The problem of function in restorative dentistry. *J Prosthet. Dent.* 1955; 5: 670.

[12] Schallhorn RG. A study of the arbitrary center and the kinematic center of rotation for face-bow mountings. *J Prosthet. Dent.* 1957; 7: 162.

[13] Page HL. some confusing concepts in articulation. *Part I. Dent Digest* 1958; 64; 71.

[14] Weinberg LA. The transverse hinge axis: real or imaginary. *J Prosthet Dent.* 1959; 9:775-87.

[15] Lauritzen AG, Bodner GH. Variation in location of arbitrary and true hinge axis points. *J Prosthet Dent* 1961; 11: 224.

[16] TrapozzanoVR, Lazzari JB. A study of hinge axis determination. *J Prosthet Dent.* 1961; 11:858.

[17] Aull AE. A study of the transverse axis. *J Prosthet. Dent.* 1963; 13:469-79.

[18] Long JH. Location of the terminal hinge axis by intra-oral means. *J Prosthet Dent.* 1970; 23: 11

[19] Hellsing G, Hellsing E, Eliasson S. The hinge axis concept: a radiographic study of its relevance. *J Prosthet Dent.* 1995; 73: 60-4.

[20] Seifert D, Jerolimov V, Carek V. Terminal hinge axis--Hobo point--Frankfurt horizontal relations. *Coll Antropol.* 2000; 24: 479-84.

[21] Bowley JF, Morgano SM. Occlusal plane discrepancies generated by transverse horizontal axis deviations. *J Prosthet Dent* 2001; 86: 67-73.

[22] Nagy WW, Smithy TJ, Wirth CG. Accuracy of a predetermined transverse horizontal mandibular axis point. *J Prosthet Dent* 2002; 87:387-94.

[23] Preston JD. A reassessment of the mandibular transverse horizontal axis theory. 1979. *J Prosthet Dent.* 2004; 91:505-12.

[24] Thieme KM, Kubein-Meesenburg D, Ihlow D, Sadat-Khonsari R, Moldovan O, Nägerl H. The mandibularly fixed hinge axis--investigation of patients with sound and pathological jaws. *Ann Anat.* 2007; 189(4):384-6.

[25] Konate NY, Djérédou KB, Kamagaté FS, Thiam A, Pesson DM, Assi KD, Touré S. Determination of the average value of the condylar slope of black Africans. *Odontostomatol Trop.* 2008 Sep;31(123):33-7.

[26] Tokiwa H, Nakazawa F, Ozaki M, Nakamura Y. Anatomical location of various condylar points for jaw movement analysis in Japanese women. *J Oral Rehabil.* 2010 Apr;37(4):235-41. Epub 2010 Jan 13.

[27] Lucia, V. O. : Centric Relation-Theory and Practice, *J. Prosthet Dent.* 1960;10: 849-56.

[28] Craddock FW, Symmons HF. Evaluation of the Face-Bow, *J. Prosthet Dent.* 1952; 2: 634.

[29] Lauritzen AG, Wolford LW. Hinge Axis Location on an Experimental Basis, *J. Prosthet Dent.* 1961; 11: 1059.

[30] Kurth LE, Feinstein IK. The Hinge Axis of the Mandible, *J. Prosthet. Dent.* 1951; 1:3. 27.

[31] Fenn HRB, Liddelow KP, Gimson AP. *Clinical Dental Prosthetics*. London: Staples Press, 1961: 274.

[32] Henderson D, Steffel V L. *McCracken's Removable Partial Prosthodontics*, 4th ed. St. Louis: The C. V. Mosby Co. ,1973: 173-74.

[33] Osborne J, Lammie G A. *Partial Dentures*, 3rd ed. Oxford and Edinburgh: Scientific Publications, 1968: 367-68.
[34] . Bergstrom G. On the reproduction of dental articulation by means of articulators, a kinematic investigation. *Acta Odontol Stand.* 1950; 9, suppl 4.
[35] Dawson PE. Evaluation, Diagnosis, and Treatment of Occlusal Problems. St. Louis: The C. V. Mosby Co. , 1974: 132-34.
[36] Abdal-Hadi L. The hinge axis: evaluation of current arbitrary determination methods and a proposal for a new recording method. *J Prosthet Dent.* 1989; 62:463-7.
[37] Lejoyeux J, *Prothese complete.* Tome 23rd ed. Paris: Maloine. S. A editeur. 1976; 223-45, 294.
[38] Razek A. Clinical evaluation of methods used in locating the mandibular hinge axis. *J Prosthet Dent.* 1981; 46:369-73.
[39] Palik JF, Nelson DR, White JT. Accuracy of an earpiece face-bow. *J Prosthet Dent.* 1985; 53:800-4.
[40] Renner RP, Lau VM. Hinge-axis location and face-bow transfer for edentulous patients. *J Prosthet Dent.* 1976; 35:352-6.
[41] Gunderson RB, Parker MH. An alternative technique for location of the hinge axis. *J Prosthet Dent.* 1987; 58:448-50.
[42] Beresin, V. E., and Schiesser, F. J.: *The Neutral Zone in Complete Dentures*, St. Louis, 1973, The C. V. Mosby Company, p. 89.
[43] Weinberg LA. An evaluation of the face-bow mounting. *J Prosthet Dent.* 1961; 11:32-42.
[44] Gillis, R. R.: Articulator development and the importance of observing the condyle paths in full denture prosthesis. *J Am Dent Assoc.* 1926; 13: 3-25.
[45] Gordon SR, Stoffer WM, Connor SA. Location of the terminal hinge axis and its effect on the second molar cusp position. *J Prosthet Dent.* 1984; 52:99-105.
[46] Walker PM. Discrepancies between arbitrary and true hinge axes. *J Prosthet Dent.* 1980; 43:279-85.

In: A Window on Surgery and Orthodontics
Editor: Giuseppe Scardina
ISBN: 978-1-62808-948-6

Chapter XI

Tissue Sculpturing: A Method for Improving Esthetics of Anterior Fixed Prosthodontics: A Clinical Report

D. R. Prithviraj*, K. M. Regish and Deeksha Sharma
Department of Prosthodontics
Government Dental College and Research Institute, Bangalore
Victoria Hospital Campus, Fort, Bangalore, India

Abstract

Esthetically correct treatment of a localized alveolar ridge defect is a frequent prosthetic challenge. Such defects can be overcome not only by a variety of prosthetic means, but also by several periodontal surgical techniques, notably soft tissue augmentations. This article describes a technique for the improvement of esthetics with conditioning of the tissue beneath the pontics. The technique describes a procedure where a free connective tissue graft is used for augmenting the localized ridge defect followed by a metal ceramic restoration enhancing the esthetics, function and comfort.

Keywords: Soft tissue augmentation, connective tissue augmentation, metal ceramic restoration, alveolar ridge defect

Introduction

Esthetics associated with health of surrounding tissues in fixed prosthodontics is arduous, especially when treating the maxillary anterior region. An unfavorable relationship between residual ridge, pontic, and gingival papilla commonly compromises the final result. The shape

* Tel: +919620204727, prithvidr@yahoo.com.

of a pontic should be designed to meet functional demands, promote access, and ensure esthetics, with the goal of maintaining the health of the adjacent tissue. For this reason, a convex tissue surface is indicated for pontics of posterior or anterior fixed partial dentures (FPDs). However, the convex shape of the residual ridge often does not allow the dentist to construct a satisfactory, well-shaped pontic. Alteration of the shape of a residual ridge by surgical intervention has been a valuable management strategy to improve tissue contour. [1]

Siebert has classified residual ridge deformities into three categories:

1. Class I defect: Faciolingual loss of tissue height and normal height of ridge.
2. Class II defect: Loss of ridge height with normal width of the ridge.
3. Class III defect: A combination of loss of both the dimensions [2, 3]

Abrams et al. studied the prevalence of anterior ridge deformities in the mandibular and maxillary arches of partially edentulous patients and reported the presence of defects in 91% of the cases. Class III defects were the most prevalent (55. 8%), followed by Class I defects (32. 8%) and Class II defects (2. 9%). [4]. Restoration with fixed partial dentures in these cases is complicated, mainly because of the esthetic complications that arise. Dark interdental spaces occur, and the pontics do not resemble natural teeth in terms of shape, height, or size. Furthermore, these devices frequently cause phonetic, eating, and oral hygiene difficulties. [5, 6]. Various techniques have been proposed to correct these tissue deformities, i. e, guided bone regeneration, bone grafts and bone substitutes below a flap or in a tunnel made in the damaged ridge area, and procedures for ridge augmentation with soft tissues. [6] Within the latter category, three main techniques have been employed:

1. Full-thickness free gingival or onlay graft using the palate as a donor area, as proposed by Seibert. [2]
2. Free subepithelial connective tissue graft implanted in a tunnel or pouch prepared in the mucosa that lines the defect, as proposed by Langer and Calagna [7] and modified by Garber and Rosenberg. [8]
3. "Roll" technique described by Abrams. [9]

This clinical report describes the soft-tissue ridge augmentation to correct Class III alveolar ridge defect combined with fixed prosthodontics to achieve maximum esthetics, comfort and function.

Clinical Report

A 35yr old male with missing left maxillary central incisor was evaluated for restorative treatment. Medical history revealed no systemic disease. Dental history revealed the loss of left maxillary central incisor following a blow in a road traffic accident 18 months back. Careful clinical and radiologic examination revealed an alveolar ridge defect in height as well as labiopalatal direction (Siebert's Class III) [2, 3] [Figure 1]. Loss of width of the bone in faciopalatal direction was more pronounced than the ridge height. A fixed partial denture

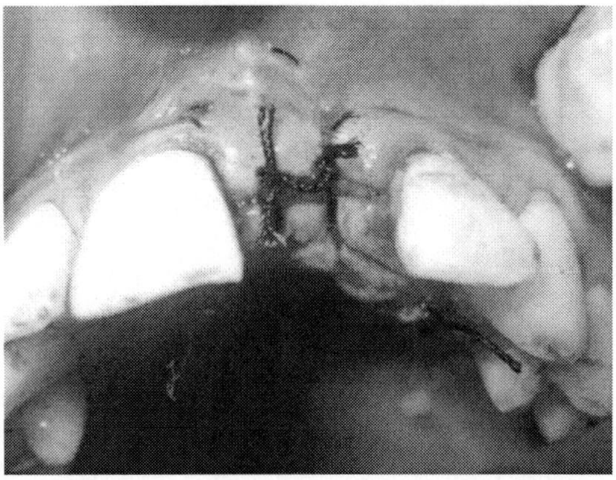

Figure 5. Connective tissue graft in place.

A eugenol dressing is placed with the help of a surgical stent, and the patient is given normal postoperative instructions. The dressing and sutures are removed after 1 week and the region is either left uncovered or redressed for an additional week. Healing was uneventful. Recall appointment were scheduled on regular basis.

Prosthodontic Treatment

Home care instructions were reviewed and the patient was recalled after 1 month for the fabrication of the prosthesis. On recall appointment the ridge form was evaluated and considered acceptable for the permanent restoration [Figure 6]. Three unit metal ceramic restoration was fabricated using right maxillary central incisor and left maxillary lateral incisor as abutment teeth to replace the maxillary left central incisor with a naturally looking pontic [Figure 7]. Recall appointment were timely scheduled again and it was noticed that there was no relapse of the augmented area and esthetics, function and comfort was adequately restored.

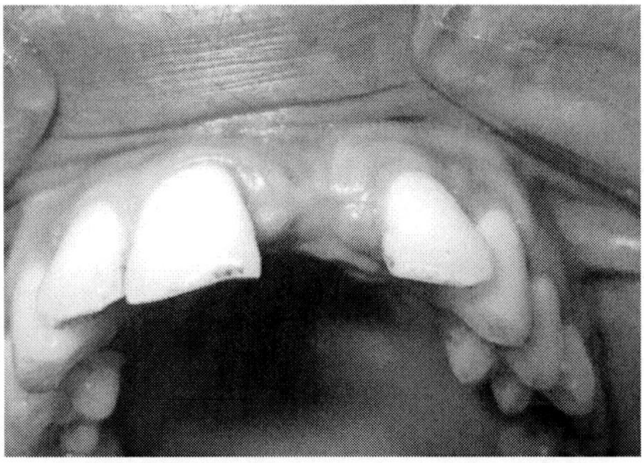

Figure 6. One month post-operative view.

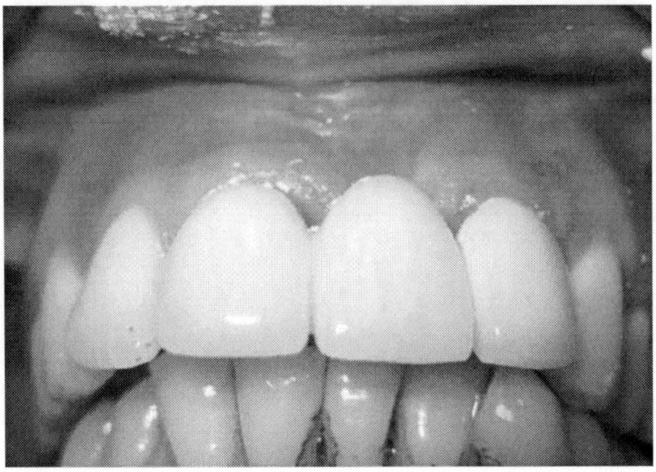

Figure 7. Metal ceramic restoration.

Discussion

Soft tissue grafts have been successfully used for many years to cover areas of alveolar ridge reconstruction. Important factors to be considered for the long-term success of free mucosal and connective tissue transplants include primary fixation of the graft, the possibility of revascularization, and revitalization from the receptor site. Close contact to a well-vascularized receptor site positively influences the prognosis of free grafts. A subepithelial connective tissue graft between the mucosa and the periosteum is more predictable and has a much better chance of survival than free grafts over poor or nonvascularized areas such as a bone graft or a nonresorbable membrane. [10]

In this case a surgical procedure was employed for augmenting the defective ridge as the optimal treatment and a metal ceramic FPD was selected as the best restorative option. After augmentation and placement of the prosthesis, the patient was examined on a 6-month recall period in which the clinical criteria for failure of treatment were evaluated, i. e. , sign of pain or discomfort, inflammation or infection, mobility of the abutment teeth, radiolucency, or radiographic detectable bone loss.

In conclusion, this clinical report suggests that soft tissue augmentation with free connective tissue graft from the palate, in conjunction with a metal ceramic FPD, is a viable treatment to provide esthetically acceptable contours to the alveolar ridge and an effective restoration.

References

[1] Jacques LB, Coelho AB, Hollweg H, Conti PC. Tissue sculpturing: an alternative method for improving esthetics of anterior fixed prosthodontics. *J. Prosthet. Dent.* 1999,81:630-3.

[2] Siebert J. Reconstruction of deformed, partially edentulous ridges, using full thickness onlay grafts. Part 1. Technique and wound healing. *Compend. Contin. Dent* 1983;4:437-53.

[3] Mishra N, Singh BP, Rao J, Rastogi P. Improving prosthetic prognosis by connective tissue ridge augmentation of alveolar ridge. *Indian J. Dent. Res.* 2010 Jul;21:129-31.

[4] Abrams H, Kopczyk R, Kaplan A. Incidence of anterior ridge deformities in partially edentulous patients. *J. Prosthet. Dent.* 1987;57: 191-4.

[5] Studer S, Naef R, Schaer P. Adjustment of localized alveolar ridge defects by soft tissue transplantation to improve mucogingival esthetics: A proposal for clinical classification and an evaluation of procedures. *Quintessence Int.* 1997;28 785-805.

[6] Gasparini DO. Double-fold connective tissue pedicle graft: a novel approach for ridge augmentation. *Int. J. Penodontics Restorative Dent.* 2004 24:280-7.

[7] Langer B, Calagna L. The subepithelial connective tissue graft. *J. Prosthet. Dent.* 1980;44:363-7.

[8] Garber D, Rosenberg E. The edentulous ridge in fixed prosthodontics. *Compend. Contin. Educ. Dent.* 1981;2:212-24.

[9] Abrans L. Augmentation of the deformed residual edentulous ridge for fixed prosthesis. *Compend. Contin. Educ. Dent.* 1980;1:205-14.

[10] Khoury F, Happe A. The palatal subepithelial connective tissue flap method for soft tissue management to cover maxillary defects: a clinical report. *lnt. J. Oral Maxillofac Implants* 2000;15:415-8.

In: A Window on Surgery and Orthodontics
Editor: Giuseppe Alessandro Scardina
ISBN: 978-1-62808-948-6

Chapter XII

Development of Root Analogue Implants – A Review Study

***D. R. Prithviraj*[1]*, *Ashu Sharma*[2], *K. M. Regish*[3], and *Deeksha Sharma*[4]**

[1]Dept. of Prosthodontics, Govt. Dental College and Research Institute, Bangalore Victoria Hospital Campus, Fort, Bangalore, India

[2]Dept. of Prosthodontics, Bangalore Institute of Dental Sciences and Hospital, Wilson Garden, Bangalore, India

[3,4]Dept. of Prosthodontics, Govt. Dental College and Research Institute, Bangalore, Victoria Hospital Campus, Fort, Bangalore, India

Abstract

Immediate placement with conventional cylindrical implants into extraction sockets has many disadvantages owing to the incongruence of the implant to the extraction socket resulting in a void adjacent to the head of the implant.

The purpose of this article is to review the developments that have taken place in root-analogue implants over years including, how various implant materials, implant fabrication and implant placement techniques for root-analogue implants have evolved with time.

Keywords: Immediate implantation, root-analogue implants, dental polymer implant, zirconia root-analogue implant, custom-made implant

* Tel:+919620204727; Email:Prithvidr@Yahoo.Com.

Introduction

Replacement of missing single tooth with implants has become everyday treatment modality in dental clinics, hospitals and academic institutions. Originally, a healing period of 6-9 months was recommended by Adell et al. [1], before implant insertion (late implant placement). Later, earlier placement of implants after only 2-3 months was proposed (delayed implant placement) by Tarnow and Fletcher [2], and more recently immediate implant placement [3, 4, 5, 6] within a few days of tooth extraction has been performed clinically, but in highly selected cases only. [7] For an implant to be placed successfully into a fresh extraction socket and also to increase its prognosis, it should have the anatomy similar to the tooth extracted. This is very important because if we place a round or cylindrical implant in an extraction socket, a void/gap is often evident between implant and the orifice of the socket due to the discrepancy in size and shape between the implant and the extraction orifice leading to its failure. [8] According to Gary Coatoam and Angelo Mariotti, a number of researchers have reported on barrier membranes or grafting materials used for the exclusion of epithelium so that bone could fill into the void. [8] However to simplify the immediate implant procedure it would be preferable to utilize root analogue implants which are of the same form and size as the extracted tooth. Such an implant would fit into extraction socket due to its congruence with the socket. [9]

Search Strategy

A PubMed search of English literature was conducted up to January 2010 using the terms: implants, immediate implantation, root-analogue implants, dental polymer implant, zirconia root-analogue implant, custom-made implant and immediate extraction socket. Additionally, the bibliographies of 7 previous reviews as well as articles published in Clinical Oral -Implants Research, International Journal of Oral and Maxillofacial Implants, International Journal of Oral and Maxillofacial surgery, International Journal of Prosthodontics, Journal of Periodontology, Journal of Oral Implantology, Journal of prosthetic dentistry, International journal of prosthodontics, Journal of dental research, International journal of periodontics and restorative dentistry were manually searched.

History

The concept of replacing teeth with custom-made root analogue implants is not new. The oldest evidence of a dental implant dates back to around 550 BC. [10, 11] In ancient times, wood, metal, shell or stone were carved and shaped to form the root for the implant. [12] The first literature reference to a modern style implant came in 1809 when Maggiolo described a tooth root-shaped implant made out of 18-carat gold. [13]

In 1969, the concept of replacing teeth with custom-made root-analogue implants was again reported; however, the autopolymerised and heat processed polymethacrylate was utilized to fabricate the tooth analogue which was encapsulated by soft tissue rather than osseointegrated. Lundgren and colleagues reintroduced the idea of root-analogue implants in 1922. Instead of using polymers, titanium was utilized in an experimental model of immediate implant placement, leading to bony integration in 88%. [14, 15] A good fit between implant and the host bed has been described as an important factor for implant success. [14, 16]. Kohal et al. further refined the approach of root-analogue titanium implants by widening the coronal aspect of the implant to compensate for the lost periodontium and to obtain a good congruence between implant and extraction socket. In several instances, the implant insertion led to fractures of the thin buccal wall of the alveolar bone. A clinical study performed by W. Pirker and A. Kocher described an excellent primary stability of root-analogue titanium implants that sustained up to 1 month, with a highly disappointing failure rate of 48% at 9 months follow-up.

A perfect fit of the implant without any retentions leads to an excellent primary stability; however, at the same time, it might be responsible for the intermediate term failure, because of the subsequent uniform pressure-induced resorption concerning the entire alveolar surface simultaneously. A cross-section of the jaws shows that there is only sufficient room for enlargements and retentions in the interdental space, whereas the thin buccal and lingual layers do not allow for any enlargement of implants in this area. [17]

In a recently developed root analogue implant system, CAD/CAM was used for the fabrication of the root analogue which allowed the immediate replacement of teeth which had to be extracted. [16, 18] Alternatively copy milling of the extracted teeth can also be done. Several authors reported the advantages of the root analogue implant. Lundgren concluded that this system osseointegrated with a high degree of predictability and the quality of bone-to-implant contact was high enough to function well. [17] However; long surgical time was needed in immediate replacement with this system.

Recently three-dimensional imaging has been developed to gather a vast number of complex slice images. [19] Instead of the traditional implantation procedure, a CT scanning of tooth could be processed and converted into root analogue implant. [20] This technological advancement was termed rapid prototyping. With rapid prototyping techniques, the surgical time can be reduced and the implant operation could be simplified. There were various subdivisions in rapid prototyping techniques. Two methods, fused deposition modeling and stereolithography are the most frequently used techniques. It is less clear; however, whether this is an accurate and reliable technique. [19]

Materials Used as Root Analogue Implants

1. Auto-polymerized and heat-processed polymethacrylate.
2. Titanium.
3. Ceramics (Aluminium oxide, Zirconia)

Dental Polymer Implant Material

Hodosh et al. (1969, 1972) introduced the dental polymer implant philosophy. Autopolymerized and heat-processed polymethacrylate was utilized to fabricate the tooth replica/analogue implants. According to the authors these implants were surrounded by a connective tissue membrane composed of collagenous fibers. Since it is the bony integration of dental implants that would lead to the most predictable long term results (Adell et al. 1981), today polymers are not used as dental implant material any more. [9]

Reasons for Use of Polymers in Implantology [21]

1. They can be 'tailor-made" to specific needs, since components can be added or deleted to change the physical characteristics of the polymers. For example, they can be made more or less porous, harder, softer, purer, etc.
2. They are easy to handle for fabrication purposes and permit accuracy of reproduction.
3. They do not emit microwaves of electrolytic current as do metals.
4. Fibrous connective tissue attachment to the polymer implants has been shown to be possible.
5. Microscopic evaluation is easier than with metals.

Autopolymerizing and heat-processed polymethacrylate, alone or combined with grated cancellous freeze-dried calf bone (an organic) are the main materials which have been used to develop the polymer implant concept. Boplant-Methacrylate implants – are methacrylate with bone embedded in it. This combination, when in proper percentages, has been used in several ways since it is biologically acceptable [22] and does not cause untoward immunologic reactions. The term polymer implant refers to polymer materials that, when combined with additives, can change their physical properties to improve their acceptance by the host for a specific purpose. The plastic or plastic-bone mixture, a material developed in the laboratory of division of health sciences at brown university, has been used successfully for the tooth replica implant. By immediately fabricating the implant, the replica of the extracted natural tooth is placed in the socket within 45 minutes after its extraction or loss.

Failures of Dental Polymer Implants [23]

1. There was high rate of mechanical failures.
2. The circumference of the implant at the area of permucosal penetration was large, since the shape of the implants was cylindrical.
3. The early failures demonstrated an extensive accumulation of chronic inflammatory cells and rapid bone loss with loosening of the implant.

Titanium Root Analogue Implant Systems
(Re-Implant System, Frialit-2 System and PACE System Implant Material)

In 1992 Lundgren and co-workers (1992) reintroduced the idea of root analogue implants. Instead of using polymers, commercially pure titanium was utilized for the fabrication of the implants [17]

Titanium has been used for making root analog implants for it best biocompatibility and osseointegration properties. Above mentioned three titanium anatomical root implant systems has been investigated so far. The advantages of these types of implant systems treatment method compared to the use of conventional cylinder or screw-type implants include improved biomechanics, easier surgical procedures, and simpler fabrication of an esthetic crown, and cheaper price. One remarkable feature of the Re Implant procedure is its simplicity, as no sophisticated surgical procedures needs to be performed. The strength of the Re- Implant system is the preservation of soft and hard tissues; the implants resemble the tooth at soft tissue level, allowing retention of the biologic contour of the soft tissue and the interdental papillae. In addition, conventional implants do not have the shape of a natural root, and therefore, difficulties in obtaining an adequate emergence profile for the final prosthesis might evolve. [24]

Ceramic Dental Implants: Tubingen Implant Material (Frialit-1 Immediate Implant)

The Tubingen implant system was developed for the immediate replacement of anterior teeth (Schulte and Heimke, 1976). The implants have dimensions that resemble the sizes of natural roots [25]. In 1984 professor W. Schulte [26] published his report on intra-osseous (Frialit-1) Tubingen implants. These implants were made up of aluminium oxide. The biophysical concept particularly anticipated immediate replacement of teeth following their extraction; this differentiates the present system from most other implant systems. In Tubingen implant system the shape of the implant is not exactly same as the root of the tooth to be extracted but it is the close approximation of it. The dentine-like colour and the biological properties of the bio-inert Al2O3 implant material is an advantage to the aesthetics of the prosthetic restorations and to the condition of the soft tissues in the permucosal area. The Tubingen implant is placed with a one-phase technique implying special care for the temporary restorations to avoid premature loading. Even when a Tubingen implant can be placed under optimal conditions regarding the quality of alveolar bone and the surrounding tissues, direct bone contact will only be possible when the implant is not loaded during at least 3 months. Advantage of the Tubingen implants and their conical root forms were the large diameters which make them suitable for the replacement of front teeth. Disadvantage of the Tubingen implant is that a one-phase implant produces the danger of possible premature initial loading which can cause loss of the implant [25].

The development of two-phase implants, with the same conical root forms, for replacement of front teeth was realized with Frialit-2 and was a subject of further studies (Schulte et al., 1992).

Zirconia as Root- Analogue Implant Material

Zirconia, which emerged as an alternative material to titanium for root-analogue dental implant fabrication, can be used because of its superior mechanical and chemical properties, improved esthetic results by preventing dark discoloration of the gum and the display of titanium roots in case of gum recession. It has a high flexural strength, compressive strength, high bending forces, good hardness, and its biocompatibility as a dental implant that osseointegrates to the same extent as titanium implants has been demonstrated in several animal investigations. [27, 28]

Finally in 2008 and 2009 W. Pirker and A. Kocher published a clinical report by selecting root-identical implants with significant modifications by using zirconia. They claimed to publish a report on first successful immediate replacement of a three rooted tooth with three rooted zirconia implant. The goal of these studies was to evaluate a novel approach to root-analogue dental implants. [7, 14]

Immediate Placement of Root-Analogue Implants

Immediate implant placement post-extraction has resulted in the initiation of prosthetic treatment in as little as 3 to 6 months, with additional benefit of reducing alveolar bone resorption. [29] One of the reasons for development of root analogue implants was to reduce the overall treatment time which was possible by immediate placement of implants after extraction of the tooth.

Indications [14]:- Immediate root analogue implants can be used best in situations where tooth is extracted due to root caries, vertical or horizontal root fracture, endodontic lesions, and unsuccessful root canal treatment. Chronic apical paradontitis is not an exclusion criterion, but in these cases the area of infection should be removed.

1. Advantages and Disadvantages of Immediate Implantation [5, 31]

ADVANTAGES	DISADVANTAGES
1. Reduction in time of therapy.	1. Lack of control of the final implant position
2. Preservation of the bone and gingival tissues.	2. Difficulty obtaining primary stability.
3. Restorative advantages:-Placement of root analogue implant fixture allows bone to be regenerated in the area previously occupied by the extracted tooth.	3. Inadequate soft tissue coverage.
4. It also maximizes the length of the implant placed because the implant must extend beyond the apex as far as possible for stability.	4. Inability to inspect all aspects of the extraction site for defects or infection.
5. Surgical advantages:- i. Tooth extraction can be performed without raising a mucoperiosteal flap; therefore the soft tissue trauma is minimized and the interdental papillae can be maintained. ii. Since no bone grafts or barrier membranes are necessary for closing intrabony defects, an uneventful healing can be expected. iii. Reduction in number of surgical interventions.	5. Difficulty in preparing the osteotomy due to bur movement (chatter) on the walls of the extraction site.

2. Design modifications of different root-analogue implants

Implant System	Design Modification	Purpose
1. Dental polymer root-analogue implant. 21	1. Implant roots with apical holes. Implant roots without apical holes. 2. Pure polymethacrylate implant, with and without foam agents. Bone-polymethacrylate implant, with and without foam agents.	1. Osseous bridge with periodontal ligament form through these premade holes. 2. a. Foaming agent used to produce greater porosity to implant root surface and facilitate penetration of connective tissues. b. Anorganice bone in polymethacrylate degrades, leaving openings for periodontal fibers insertion
2. Titanium Root-analogue implant	***1. Re-Implant system 31:-*** a. Honeycomb pattern. b. Root surface sandblasted and acid etched. c. Attachment of insertion bar to root implant.	a. To increase the surface area. b. To increase microretention. c. To assist dentist in implant insertion into tooth socket without touching implant root surface.
	2. PACE,CAL-Form implant system8:-	
	a. Series of premade anatomically shape implants.	a. Their shape and size corresponds to that of the osteotomes used for shaping and enlarging the osteotomy site.
	b. The anatomically shaped implant has an external bevel around the outer edge at the opening of the implant.	b. Final restoration is finished over this bevel.
	c. Two types of surgical caps:- i. Flat surgical cover. ii. Dual winged surgical caps	c. i. Allows the gingival tissue to be sutured over the head of the implant during two stage healing If left exposed, it results in a modified one-stage procedure. ii. Facilitate surgical positioning of the flaps during traditional one-stage implant placement.
	3. Frialit-232:- a. Stepped screw implant with angled abutment and straight abutment. b. Mirror polished transgingival portion.	a. Steps are made to achieve force transfer to the bone as well as possible. b. Marginal gingiva and epithelium are placed here.
3. Tubingen root-analogue implant26 (Al2O3)	1. Stepped cylinder or oval implant shapes. 2. Circular groove.	1. All rounded steps help to achieve force transfer to the bone as well as possible. 2. Marginal gingival border and its internal epithelial seam is placed into it.
(Frialit-1)	3. Lacunae on outer surface of root implant	3. To increase the surface area of contact and to reduce the pressure
4. Zirconia root-analogue implant. 14	1. Microretention on entire root surface can be done by sandblasting or acid etching. 2. Macro-retentions, strictly limited to the interdental space. 3. Reduced diameter of the implant by 0. 1- 0. 5mm next to the thin cortical bone.	1. To get beyond primary stability and improve osseointegration beyond the period of 1 month and bone remodeling 2. To avoid fracture and pressure-induced bone loss.

Contraindications [30]:- Immediate root analogue implants are not recommended in cases with severe labial and circumferential bone defects, bony defects with two or three missing walls, horizontal defects of more than 1. 5 mm.

Designs and Modifications

Root analogue implant designs have evolved over time with the change in materials used for their fabrication. These modifications in their designs were done to improve their mechanical properties and also to promote better initial stability and rapid osseointegration with the surrounding bone. These modifications included changes in surface topography and diameter of implant.

Methods of Root Analogue Implant Fabrication

Dental Polymer Root Analogue Implant Fabrication [21]

The tooth replica implant is fabricated in the following manner. The natural tooth requiring extraction is removed and any defect is corrected with wax. A mold is made by investing the corrected natural tooth in stone or plaster using a flask. When multirooted teeth are to be reproduced, thin-bodied heat-resistant silicone is used. It is best applied by using an injection gun with the silicone directed into the inner trifurcation or bifurcation sections of the roots. Strands of silicone are placed to extend through the root areas so that, when the tooth with silicone attached is invested vertically in a flask, the hardened plaster will anchor the silicone when the natural tooth is removed from the finished mold and the silicone is not displaced. The implant material is test packed with very little excess, for large excess causes the implant to elongate when silicone is used. Once heat cured, the flask is cooled and opened, and the implant is finished, sandblasted, and compared with the natural tooth for accuracy of shape and size. It is placed into zephirin chloride for approximately 10 minutes, and then inserted into the alveolar socket. The implant is then splinted to adjacent teeth or implants.

Initially it was made of pure heat-processed polymethacrylate. It was later made of grated anorganic bone (cancellous) and heat-processed polymethacrylate. Bone was incorporated into the mixture since it was known to have a chemical composition similar to cementum. The polymethacrylate is nondegrading for it is not broken down by animal cells, whereas anorganic bone degrades, leaving openings into which the periodontal fibers may insert more easily resulting in gradual strengthening of the periodontal attachment to the implant.

Titanium Root Analogue Implant Fabrication

Copy-Milling Technique [17]

In year 1992 Lundgren et al. reintroduced the idea of root analogue implants. They used titanium to fabricate the implants by copy- milling techniques which were placed in beagle dog.

CAD/CAM System [31]

Also known as "Re-Implant System" for immediate placement of implants. The Re Implant system, a recently developed root analogue implant system allows the immediate replacement of teeth which have to be extracted because of decay, trauma, and internal or external resorption. It is also possible to replace multirooted teeth by splitting them into single-rooted teeth. Tooth replacement with the Re Implant system is contraindicated in cases with extensive periodontal disease.

As described by Strub JR et al. [31] the Re Implant system is composed of a titanium milling unit with an integrated laser and a computer control station with a built-in axis control card, which is attached to the milling machine. The laser permits the touchless recording of distances against different objects and works according to the triangular principle. With special software, the data from the scanned object can be manipulated in the computer unit. The material used for the Re Implant implants is titanium grade II, which is accepted by the American Dental Association as implant material and also has the approval of the European Community (EC). The raw material is provided as prefabricated cylindrical titanium blanks of different diameters, with integrated threads for the attachment of conical abutments. With the software program, it is possible to change the dimensions and the surface characteristics of the final implant. The scanned root model dimensions are increased, so that the final implant is slightly larger than the original root. The enlargement is for compensating the compression of the alveolar bone during the extraction process and the loss of the periodontal ligament. It is needed for the primary stability of the implant. The altered computer data are transferred back to the milling unit. The two servomotors work according to the data, and the anatomic root analogue implant is fabricated out of the titanium blank, under permanent cooling.

Tubingen Implant Fabrication [25]

These implants were supplied as premade implants by the manufacturer with different sizes to approximately fit into the extraction sockets of different types of teeth. Tubingen, Frialit, implants consisted of Al_2O_3-ceramic. The shape of the Tubingen implant is basically that of a stepped cone, formed by cylinders of different diameters. The implants are available with diameters of 4, 5, 6 and 7 mm; these sizes are related to the widest cylinders of the implant.

Zirconia Root-Analogue Implant Fabrication [7]

They can be fabricated either by copy-milling technique or by CAD/CAM technique. The extracted tooth is cleaned. The root is laser scanned and macroretentions are designed that is strictly limited to the interdental space only, sparing the buccal and lingual face, to prevent fractures at the time point of insertion of the thin cortical bone layer. In addition a crown stump is designed for later connection to the crown. The implant is now milled from a medical grade zirconium dioxide block and the surface roughened by sandblast and sintered for 8 h to achieve the desired mechanical properties. Then the implant is cleaned in an ultrasonic bath containing 96% ethanol for 10 min, packaged and sterilized in a steam sterilizer. In a clinical case report reported by Kohal and Klaus regarding placement of zirconia implant immediately after extraction, a custom-made zirconia dental implant was used. The implant was fabricated ad modum ReImplant. Briefly, after having evaluated the radiographs (panoramic view, conventional tomograms), a copy of the final implant was reconstructed using selfcuring acrylic resin. This copy was mounted into the ReImplant scanning unit and scanned. The acrylic resin copy was then exchanged for a highly isostatic pressed zirconia cylinder. According to the scanning data, a high-speed handpiece incorporated into the ReImplant milling unit cut the final implant out of the zirconia cylinder. [33]. In an investigation by Kohal, Klaus and Strub to test zirconia implants restored with different all-ceramic crowns with the titanium implant serving as control, an extracted maxillary central left incisor served as a model for the fabrication of the titanium and zirconia implants. The root was transformed into a titanium implant using the ReImplants Unit. Commercially pure titanium grade 2 was used as implant material. The tooth root was scanned by the system immanent laser, and the obtained data were stored in the computer unit of the system. Then, the tooth root was replaced by a cylindrical titanium blank and the milling unit processed the implant according to the computer data. For the ceramic implants, prefabricated partially stabilized zirconia cylinders with a length of 20mm and a diameter of 10mm were used. The titanium implant model obtained from the ReImplants Unit was copied into a zirconia implant using the Celays System. [34]

Methods of Root Analogue Implant Placement

Except for some modifications, discussed below, the implant placement procedures are almost same for all the materials used for root analogue implants.

Zirconia Root Analogue Implant Placement [7]

The compromised tooth should be carefully extracted under local anesthesia, avoiding damage to the socket and soft tissue. The extraction socket was cleaned meticulously by means of curettage and iodoform soaked cotton gauze is placed in the socket in the mean time the implant is fabricated. Few hours or days, after extraction the iodoform cotton gaze is removed. The alveolar socket again is curetted and flushed with sterile physiologic saline solution. The custom-made individualized implant is then placed into the socket under finger pressure and subsequent gentle tapping with a hammer and a mallet. Primary stability is achieved and checked by palpation and percussion. The patient receives postoperative analgesics on demand and antibiotic medication for 4 days.

Patient is instructed to chew predominantly on the contralateral side and avoid hard food. At the control visit 10 days later the site is checked for clinically healthy marginal area and for postoperative pain or swelling. [7]

Dental Polymer Implant Placement [21]

Procedure Is Almost Same Except That

1. During polymer implant placement, an undercut preparation is made in the adjacent tooth crown to provide an attachment point for a fixation splint.
2. The polymer implant is immediately fabricated after tooth extraction and is placed in the socket within 45 minutes after tooth extraction or loss.
3. The final position of the implant is such that the junction of crown and root is 1mm below the bony crest. Mucosa is trimmed as necessary to adapt closely and sutured firmly around implant.
4. A tightly fitting rubber dam is placed over the adjacent tooth and implant, and a cold cure Polymethymethacrylate (PMMA) splint is constructed.

Titanium Implant Placement

Re-Implant Implant Placement [24]

Procedure is same except that on the following day after extraction, under local anesthesia, the apical extension is prepared under internal cooling with sterile saline solution with 2- and 3-mm titanium twist drills (Re-Implant) using the drilling stent, which is held in place with a forceps. The Re-Implant implant is then placed into the socket.

PACE implant system [8]: Following are the variations in the procedure:

1. In this implant system, oval osteotomes are successively inserted into the extraction orifice to determine the head size of the appropriate implant.
2. The oval osteotomes correspond exactly in size to the head of the implant fixtures. The proper head size is determined when the osteotome begins to bind in the opening of the tooth socket and requires gentle but deliberate force to be inserted to 1 mm above the level of the crestal bone.
3. Radiographs and direct measurements within the socket are used to determine the length of the implant. Additional sound bone is often found apical to the tip of the socket, and the depth of the osteotomy site may be increased to utilize this support.
4. In order to prevent binding of the implant, a counter bevel cannon drill may be used to hone the sides of the osteotomy site prior to implant insertion. Once the osteotomy site had been developed, the implant is transferred to the site.

Frialit-1 (Aluminium Oxide) Implant Placement [25]

1. Wijs et al. in 1994 carried out a study on Tubingen implants and described their procedure for Tubingen implant placement.
2. According to them, a full flap can be prepared to inspect the quality and quantity of the buccal part of the alveolar bone.
3. Bone preparation is executed with slow speed high torque rotation equipment (300-700 rpm).
4. The direction of the preparation is shifted to the palatal direction to avoid perforation of the buccal cortical bone at the apical side, while the pressure of the drill at the same time is also in oral direction to prevent damage of the alveolar arch.

Conclusion and Summary

The single-tooth implant placement with immediate root analogue implants is a viable treatment modality for replacing a single tooth in patients in whom adjacent teeth do not have caries or restorations, bone quantity and trabeculation are adequate, esthetics are not compromised and occlusion/function dictates can be addressed. [35] Root analogue implantology has come a long way. It all began with Polymethymethacrylate (polymer implants), then came the Aluminium oxide (Tubingen) and Titanium (Re-Implant and Frialit-2) root analogue implants. Currently, zirconia root-analogue implants are being investigated for their better mechanical and esthetical properties.

The root-analogue implantology has evolved not only in terms of the materials being used but also in the different methods that are available for the fabrication with the same material. Methods of fabrication have evolved from polymerization [21, 22] (polymer implants) to copy-milling [17] to computer aided design and milling [9, 33] (CAD/CAM) to pre-fabricated anatomically shaped [8] dental implants.

As the field of root-analogue implantology is progressing, so are the modifications made in designs of the implants to improve their stability and osseointegration with the surrounding bone and the new therapies for immediate tooth replacement continue to develop. However, the predictability and success of these procedures will need to be evaluated for immediate and long-term success.

References

[1] Adell R, Lekholm U, Rockler B, Brånemark PI. A 15-year study of osseointegrated implants in the treatment of the edentulous jaw. *Int. J. Oral Surg.* 1981 Dec;10(6):387-416.

[2] Tarnow D, Fletcher P. The 2 to 3 month post-extraction placement of root form implants: a useful compromise. *Implant: Cli. Rev. Dent.* 1993;2:l-8.

[3] Tolman DE, Keller EE. Endosseous implant placement immediately following dental extraction and alveoloplasty: preliminary report with 6-year follow-up. *Int. J. Oral Maxillofac Implants*. 1991;6(1):24-8.

[4] Barzilary I. Gaser GN, Caton J, Shenkle G. Immediate implantation of pure titanium threaded implants into extraction sockets. J. Dent. Res. 1988; 67(Spec Issue): 234.

[5] Lazzara RJ. Immediate implant placement into extraction sites: surgical and restorative advantages. *Int. J. Periodontics Restorative Dent.* 1989;9(5):332-43.

[6] Kohal RJ, Klaus G, Gieloff B, Hurzeler MB. Strub JR. Root analogue titanium implants for immediate implant placement. The Re Implant System. *Pract. Periodont. Aesthet. Dent.* 1997. (In press).

[7] Pirker W, Kocher A: Immediate, non-submerged, root-analogue zirconia implant in single tooth replacement. *Int. J. Oral Maxillofac. Surg*. 2008; 37: 293–5.

[8] Coatoam GW, Mariotti A. Immediate placement of anatomically shaped dental implants. *J. Oral Implantol*. 2000;26(3):170-6.

[9] Kohal RJ, Hurzeler MB, Mota LF, Klaus G, Caffesse RG, Strub JR. Custom-made root analogue titanium implants placed into extraction sockets. An experimental study in monkeys. *Clin. Oral Impl. Res.* 1997;8:386-392.

[10] Allen C. *Curious observations on the teeth.* John Bale, Sons and Danielsson, LTD 1987:12-13.

[11] Atilla G. A rare find in Anatolia--a tooth implant (mid-sixth century B. C.). *J. Oral Implantol.* 1993;19(1):54-7.

[12] Asbell MB. *Dentistry: A historical perspective.* Bryn Mawr: Penn. Dorrance-Company, Inc 1988:45-60.

[13] Becker MJ. Ancient "dental implants": a recently proposed example from France evaluated with other spurious examples. *Int. J. Oral Maxillofac Implants.* 1999;14(1):19-29.

[14] Pirker W, Kocher A: Immediate, non-submerged, root-analogue zirconia implants placed into single-rooted extraction sockets: 2-year follow-up of a clinical study. *Int. J. Oral Maxillofac. Surg.* 2009; 38: 1127–32.

[15] Carlsson L, Röstlund T, Albrektsson B, Albrektsson T. Removal torques for polished and rough titanium implants. *Int. J. Oral Maxillofac Implants* 1988;3:21–4.

[16] Kohal RJ, Heydecke G, Mota LF, Klaus G, Caffesse RG, Strub JR. Custom made root analogue titanium implants placed into extraction sockets. *Clin. Oral Impl. Res.* 1997;8:386-92.

[17] Lundgren D, Rylander H, Andersson M, Johansson C, Albrektson T. Healing-in of root analog titanium implants placed in extraction sockets. An experimental study in the beagle dog. *Clin. Oral Implant Res.* 1992;3:136–144.

[18] Beagle JR. The Immediate Placement of Endosseous Dental Implants in Fresh Extraction Sites. *Dent. Clin. North Am.* 2006;50(3):375-89.

[19] Lee-Ra Cho, Chang-Jin Park, In-Woo Park. A study on the dimensional accuracy of models using 3-dimensional computer tomography and 2 rapid prototyping methods. *J Korean Acad. Prosthodont.* 2001;39 (6):633-40.

[20] Schmitt SM, Chance DA. Fabrication of titanium implant-retained restorations with nontraditional machining techniques. *Int. J. Prosthodont* 1995;8:332-6.

[21] Hodosh M, Povar M, Shklar G. The dental polymer implant concept. *J. Prosthet Dent.* 1969;22(3):371-80.

[22] Hodosh M., Povar M., and Shklar, G.: The Anatomic Anorganic Bone-Polymethacrylate Endosteal Dental Implant. *Oral Surg. Oral Med. Oral Pathol.* 1968 Jun;25(6):883-8.

[23] Peterson LJ, Pennel BM, McKinney RV Jr, Klawitter JJ, Weinstein AM. Clinical, radiographical, and histological evaluation of porous rooted polymethylmethacrylate dental implants. *J. Dent Res.* 1979;58(1):489-96.

[24] Heydecke G, Kohal R, Gläser R. Optimal esthetics in single-tooth replacement with the Re-Implant system: a case report. *Int. J. Prosthodont.* 1999;12(2):184-9.

[25] De Wijs FL, Van Dongen RC, De Lange GL, De Putter C. Front tooth replacement with Tübingen (Frialit) implants. *J. Oral Rehabil.* 1994;21(1):11-26.

[26] Schulte W. The intra-osseous Al2O3 (Frialit) Tuebingen Implant. Developmental status after eight years (I-III). *Quintessence Int* 1984;15:1.

[27] Kohal RJ, Weng D, Bächle M, Strub JR. Loaded custom-made zirconia and titanium implants show similar osseointegration: an animal experiment *J. Periodontol.* 2004;75(9):1262-8.

[28] Kosmac T, Oblak C, Jevnikar P, Funduk N, Marion L. Strength and reliability of surface treated Y-TZP dental ceramics. *Inc. J. Biomed. Mater. Res.* (Appl Biomater) 2000: 53: 304–313.

[29] Gelb DA: Immediate implant surgery: three-year retrospective evaluation of 50 consecutive cases. *Int. J. Oral Maxillofac Implants* 1993;8:388-399.

[30] Bhola M, Neely AL, Kolhatkar S. Immediate implant placement: clinical decisions, advantages, and disadvantages. *J Prosthodont.* 2008 Oct;17(7):576-81. Epub 2008 Aug 26.

[31] Strub JR, Kohal RJ, Klaus G, Ferraresso F. The Re Implant System for immediate implant placement. *J. Esthet. Dent.* 1997; 9(4):187–196.

[32] Gomez-Roman G, Kruppenbacher M, Weber H, Schulte W. Immediate postextraction implant placement with root-analog stepped implants: surgical procedure and statistical outcome after 6 years. *Int. J. Oral Maxillofac Implants*. 2001;16(4):503-13.

[33] Kohal RJ, Klaus G. A zirconia implant-crown system: a case report. *Int J Periodontics Restorative Dent.* 2004 Apr;24(2):147-53.

[34] Kohal RJ, Klaus G, Strub JR. Zirconia-implant-supported all-ceramic crowns withstand long-term load: a pilot investigation. *Clin. Oral Implants Res.* 2006 Oct.;17(5):565-71.

[35] Meffert RM. Issues related to single-tooth implants. *J. Am. Dent. Assoc.* 1997;128(10):1383-90.

In: A Window on Surgery and Orthodontics
Editor: Giuseppe Alessandro Scardina
ISBN: 978-1-62808-948-6

Chapter XIII

Static Magnetic Field of Commercial Samarium-Cobalt (SmCo5) Orthodontic Magnets and DNA Fragmentation of Human Lymphocyte Cells

***Hussam M. Abdel-Kader*[1*]*, Mohamed I. Aref*[2] *and Sedky W. Yousef*[3]
[1]Faculty of Dental Medicine, AlAzhar University and Misr International University, Cairo, Egypt
[2]Faculty of Medicine, AlAzhar University, Cairo, Egypt
[3]Orthodontic Department, Faculty of Oral and Dental Medicine Misr International University (MIU), Cairo, Egypt

Abstract

Objective: The current study aimed to investigate the biological effects of the static magnetic fields of commercially available orthodontic samarium-cobalt (SmCo5) magnets on cultured human lymphocyte cells.

Materials and methods: To study the effect of the static magnetic field, in attraction and repelling modes, on human lymphocyte cells, two couples of orthodontic magnets were used. One couple was fixed with the magnets in attraction mode and the second one; the two magnets were fixed in repelling mode. On the other hand, three autoclaved glass laboratory tubes were prepared and filled with cultured human lymphocyte cells. One tube was used as a control sample and the other two were used as test samples. Each couple of the prepared orthodontic magnets was threaded into silk thread, immersed and positioned exactly in the center of the cultured lymphocytes. Modified comet assay was used to evaluate the biological effects of exposing the human lymphocyte cells for 48

* Corresponding author:Prof. Hussam M. Abdel-Kader, Professor of Orthodontics; Mena Garden City 12582; Villa B25, Louvre; 6 October City; 6 October, Egypt; E-mail: hmkader@hotmail.com; Cell phone: +2010-1189-148.

hours to the static magnetic field of orthodontic magnets under repelling and attraction modes.

Results: 1. The percentage of DNA fragmented human lymphocyte cells recorded statistically significant level ($P \leq 0.001$) after exposure for 48 hours to the static magnetic field of orthodontic magnets. 2. The adverse biological effects of the static magnetic field in attraction mode were significantly higher than that recorded in magnets' repelling mode.

Conclusion: 1. Short time exposure (48 hours) of human lymphocyte cells to the static magnetic field of the commercially used orthodontic samarium-cobalt ($SmCo_5$) magnets will end with significant DNA fragmentation of those cells. 2. The static magnetic field of magnets fixed in attraction mode has significantly higher adverse biological effects compared to that fixed in repelling mode. 3. Iron is important dynamic to augment that effect.

Keywords: Orthodontics, Orthodontic magnets, Static magnetic field, DNA fragmentation, human lymphocyte cells

Introduction

Recently, orthodontic magnets have been commercially available for clinical use and directed towards maxillary molar distalization, correction of open bite, canine retraction, fixed retention, arch expansion, functional appliances and orthodontic eruption of unerupted teeth [1-11]. Rare earth magnets made from samarium-cobalt ($SmCo_5$) or neodymium-iron-boron ($Nd_2Fe_{14}B$), are the magnets of clinical choice. Magnets readily corrode in the oral environment if they are not protected [12], and an in-vitro study revealed that unprotected orthodontic magnets, exhibited weight loss of about 31. 15% in 25 days [13]. However, in a clinical study, orthodontic magnets showed significant weight loss of about 3. 07% within six months following the loss of a protective acrylic coat within the first month of clinical use. This was accompanied by a significant release of nickel, chromium and ferrous ions [14] as well as significant apoptotic-DNA fragmentation in the patient's cheek mucosa cells. .

The adverse biological effect of $SmCo_5$ magnets in clinical use on the oral mucosa cells is a matter of debate. This could be the end results of the released metal corrosion product from the magnets after peeled-off their resin protecting coats especially nickel, cobalt and samarium and/or the effects of their static magnetic fields. The biological effect of the static magnetic field of the magnets was considered by many investigators [15-20]. The effects could be in the form of changes in cell metabolism, structure and growth. When magnets are used in orthodontics, the oral tissues will be exposed to the static magnetic field during the course of their use. The tissues, which were closest to the magnets, are supposed to be the tissues exposed significantly to the static magnetic field, than the other intraoral tissues in descending orders.

The point of interest is that orthodontic magnets are used in couple; accordingly is the biological effects of the static magnetic field the same in the repelling mode as in the attracting mode? The question is which one could have the stronger biological effects, the scattered magnetic field of repelling magnets or the combined magnetic field of attracting magnets? In the literature it is concluded that, the static magnetic field exposure value for attractive magnets is somewhat higher compared to that of repelling magnets, but the extent of the static magnetic field is wider in case of repelling magnets compared to attracting magnets [21]. In this very interesting study on the extent and flux density of the static magnetic field of samarium cobalt orthodontic magnets the authors concluded that: 1. The maximum flux density was recorded at the magnets poles. 2. Magnets in attractive mode have a flux density of 2. 2 Kg. 3. Magnets in repelling mode have a flux density of 1. 7 Kg. 4. With increased distance from the magnets the flux density decreased rapidly. Finally they reached a final conclusion that "the static magnetic field exposure of surrounding tissues can be assumed to be low, and the conceivable risk of harmful biological effects must be regarded as small and limited when the tested orthodontic magnets are used clinically".

In view of the above illustrated review of literature, the current study was directed to test the hypothesis that; the static magnetic field of commercial orthodontic magnets could have adverse biological effects on the living cells.

Materials and Methods

In the current study the biological effect of static magnetic field of commercial orthodontic magnets on cultured human lymphocyte vital cells was evaluated according to the following protocol:

1. As we commonly used orthodontic magnets in couple in different clinical orthodontic purposes, new couples of Samarium-cobalt (SmCo5) orthodontic magnets (Ortho Organizer, Inc. 424-200 Magnetic Force System) were used in the current study. In one couple, the orthodontic magnets were fixed in repelling mode (S-S poles); on the other hand, the second couple the magnets was fixed in attractive mode (S-N poles). The distance between the two magnets in the two conditions (repelling and attraction) was kept at 1. 5mm, as they are used clinically. As we used new orthodontic magnets, in the current study, with completely intact protective layer, there is no fear from the effect of metal ion release on our results.
2. Sample of heparinised human blood was collected from one of the authors (volunteered). The donor was a healthy, non-smoking 26 years old male had not been exposed to radiation, vaccinated or under medication for at least one year before the study. The collected venous blood sample had been collected under strict sterile conditions in test tubes containing heparin as anticoagulant.
3. The lymphocyte cells were separated and cultured in RBMI media contains 20% fetal calfe serum. Ferric salt in the form of Iron Dextran Complex 50 mg (10 micrometers had been used) was added as a source of iron to the cultured media [22, 23].
4. Three autoclaved laboratory glass tubes were prepared and filled with the cultured media (RBMI) contain lymphocyte cells. One tube was used as a control sample (without magnets), and the other two tubes (with magnets) were used as test samples.
5. Each couple of the prepared magnets, after autoclaving for sterilization, was threaded to silk thread and immersed and positioned exactly in the center of the cultured lymphocyte cells.
6. The three tubes were stored in an incubator at fixed temperature of C37 degrees for 48 hours.

7. Samples of the cultured lymphocyte cells were collected from the three tubes after the 48 hours test period to assess the effect of the static magnetic field on the cultured lymphocyte cells, under repelling and attraction modes compared with the control sample.
8. The potential cytotoxic and genotoxicity effects of static magnetic field of orthodontic magnets, under the two conditions, repelling-and attractive modes, on the cultured lymphocyte cells were evaluated. The severity of the case was estimated according to the percentage of apoptotic-DNA fragmented cells in the examined field.
9. Identification of the DNA fragmentation of the cultured human lymphocyte cells associated with apoptosis; was assessed by modified Comet assay technique [14].

- Stock solution (reagent): 1mg of fluorescent Ethidium bromide was added to 10 ml of PBS (phosphate buffer saline) solution.
- Preparation of the working solution: 1μL of stock solution was added into 100μL of PBS solution.
- Testing procedure: 10μL of fluorescent Ethidium bromide solution was added to cell suspension and left for one hour. The cells then were washed three times (triple wash) with the PBS solution for five minutes using centrifugation at 1000 rpm. The last centrifugation discarded the supernatant and the deposits were added to microscopic slides and glass cover-slips were used to insure even distribution and then analyzed with a fluorescent microscope using high power image (10x40).
- Detection: apoptotic cells can be discriminated by membrane blobbing and observation of the nuclear changes (swelling, loss of stain or DNA fragmentation non-fluorescent cells).
- Saving the image results; Microscopic photographic images were captured, optimized and saved using a Spot RT camera running MetaVue software under a Nikon Eclipse E400 light microscope. A 100X image was first acquired for each slide to show the entire cells. Then each image was further captured at 400X. Calculation of one hundred cells was made by the light lamb and the number of non-stained cells with the fluorescent Ethidium bromide (apoptotic changes cells; swelling, loss of stain or DNA fragmentation) was made between the one hundred cells and estimated as a percentage of DNA fragmented cells out of 100 total cells in the same field. At the time of image capture, two 400x images were saved: one for detailed assessment of normal cell (fluorescent cells) and one for detailed assessment of DNA fragmented cell.

NB: 1. The above mentioned experiment were repeated 9 times according to the same designed standard protocol.

2. For about three months several pilot studies had been undertaken till the above mentioned designs was reached and a standardized protocol for the experiment proved to be valid for the current research design.

3. During the pilot study it was noticed that magnetic field per-se had no significant effect on the cultured lymphocytes cells.

On the other hand, it was found that adding traces amount of ferrous ions to the cells' culture medium enhance the effects of the static magnetic field of orthodontic magnets on the cultured cells.

Accordingly Ferric salt in the form of Iron Dextran Complex 50 mg (10 micrometer had been used) was added as a source of iron to the cultured media [22].

Statistical Analysis

The collected data were tabulated and statistically analyzed using the following tests; Descriptive statistics (means and standard deviation) for the percentages of apoptotic-DNA fragmented human lymphocyte cells under repelling-and attractive modes was done.

Paired t test was used to test the level of statistical significant difference between the mean percentage of DNA fragmented cells before exposure to the static magnetic field and that reported after 48 hours exposure. Probabilities of less than 5% ($P \leq 0.\ 05$) were considered to be statistically significant.

Results

The pilot studies in the current study revealed that the static magnetic field of commercial orthodontic magnets in common clinical orthodontic uses, per-se, had no adverse biological effects on the cultured human lymphocyte cells. On the other hand adding traces of iron in the form of ferric salt to the culture media enhance the adverse biological effects of orthodontic magnets galvanic field on the cultured cells.

Figure 1 A and B illustrated the differences between fluorescent vital human lymphocyte cells (their nucleus were stained with Ethidium bromide) and non-fluorescent DNA fragmented cells respectively.

We can notice the different apoptotic changes of the lymphocyte cells, in the form of loss of stain of their nucleus (DNA fragmentation), swelling and complete loss of cell wall. Regarding the human lymphocyte cells, in the control sample group (without magnets) the number of vital fluorescent lymphocyte cells among the counted 100 cells, decreased significantly after the 48 hours experimental period compared to the DNA fragmented lymphocytes non-fluorescent cells (Figure 2 A and B).

On the other hand exposing the human lymphocyte cells to the static magnetic filed of commercially available orthodontic magnets for 48 hours, showed significant drop in the number of vital lymphocyte cells compared to the significant increases in DNA fragmentation of the cultured lymphocyte cells under the two conditions, attraction and-repelling mode (Figures 3 A and B respectively) compared with that of the 48 hours control sample (Figure 2 B).

The number of DNA fragmented lymphocyte cells resulting from exposure to the static magnetic field of orthodontic magnets for 48 hours was significantly higher under attractive mode compared to that in case of repelling magnets.

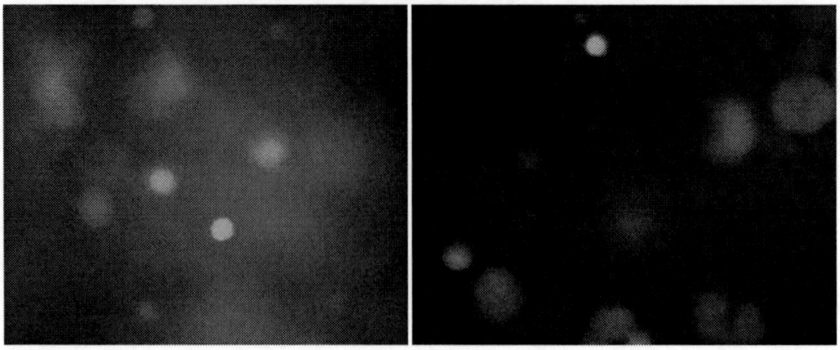

A B

Figure 1. Figure 1 A and B illustrates very few vital lymphocyte cells with intact cell wall and nucleus stained with Ethidium Bromide (fluorescent cells), on the other hand the DNA fragmented cells (non-fluorescent cells) lost their nucleus and cell wall. (Original magnification X400).

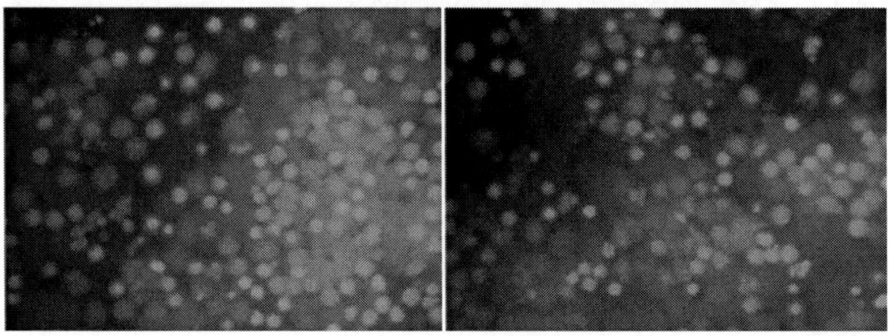

A B

Figure 2. A and B (control samples) illustrates human vital lymphocyte cells distribution in the field at the zero point and after 48 hours experimental period respectively. We can notice the increase in the number of DNA fragmented lymphocyte cells (non-fluorescent cells) after 48 hours. (Original magnification X400).

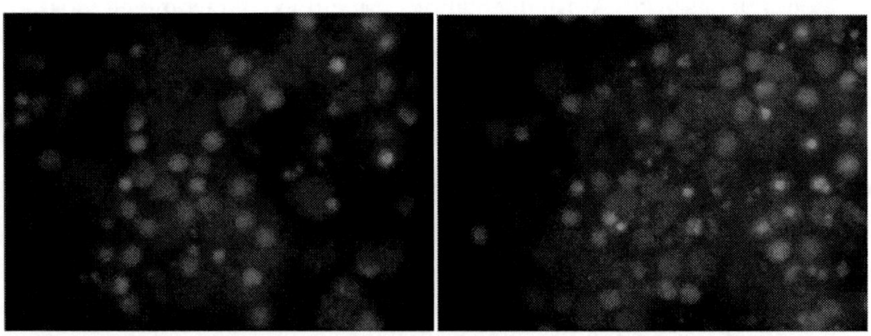

A B

Figure 3. A and B (test samples) illustrate the number of vital lymphocyte cells (fluorescent cells) compared with DNA fragmented cells (non-fluorescent cells) after 48 hours exposure to the static magnetic field arranged in attraction mode and repelling mode respectively. We can notice that the number of DNA fragmented lymphocyte cells is significantly higher in the case of attraction magnets mode compared to repelling magnets mode. (Original magnification X400).

Table 1. Descriptive statistics of the number vital human lymphocytes cells under the three conditions after the 48 hours experimental period; without magnets and after exposure to the static magnetic field of orthodontic magnets in attraction and repelling mode and the level of significant difference between changes in the three condition was evaluated using paired t test (P ≤ 0. 001)

Control group; number of vital lymphocyte cells counted among 100 cells without magnets (N=9)	1st Test sample group; number of vital lymphocyte cells counted among 100 cells with magnets at attraction mode (N=9)	2nd Test sample group; number of vital lymphocyte cells counted among 100 cells with magnets at repelling mode (N=9)	
Mean+/-SD	Mean+/-SD	Mean+/-SD	
56. 22+/-0. 7	31. 22+/-2. 82	22. 89+/-1. 29	
	Control - Attraction	Control – Repelling	Attraction - Repelling
Mean diff+/-SD diff	25. 0+/-7. 73	33. 33+/-8. 37	8. 92+/-3. 27
	t = 9. 70 P ≤ 0. 001	t = 11. 95 P ≤ 0. 001	t = 8. 18 P ≤ 0. 001

The percentage of the vital fluorescent human lymphocyte cells counted among 100 cells compared with the DNA fragmented lymphocyte cells, after 48 hours exposure to the static magnetic field of orthodontic magnets in repelling and attraction modes were evaluated. It was clearly noticed that the percentage of the vital fluorescent human lymphocyte cells decreased significantly (P ≤ 0. 001) after exposure to the static magnetic field of orthodontic magnets for only 48 hours compared to the DNA fragmented lymphocyte cells which showed dramatic increases.

These theatrical changes were significantly higher in the magnets attraction mode compared with that in repelling magnets mode where p≤0. 001 (Table 1).

Discussion

In the current study the effect of the static magnetic field of orthodontic magnets, per se, had no adverse biological effects on human living cultured lymphocyte cells. On the other hand, adding traces of iron to the medium significantly enhance DNA fragmentation of the cultured cells even after short term exposure to the static magnetic filed (48 hours). The most important finding of the current study is that; the static magnetic field of orthodontic magnets fixed in attraction mode on human lymphocyte cells, was much more destructive than that of magnets fixed in repelling mode.

Human lymphocyte cell destruction was in the form of DNA fragmentation which reached comparatively higher percentage in attraction magnets mode compared to that recorded in the case of repelling magnets condition. Our results is in accordance with that of Bondemark et al. [21] in which they concluded that; the static magnetic fields exposure values for attractive magnets were somewhat higher compared to that of repelling magnets, but the extent of the static magnetic fields is wider in case of repelling magnets compared to attracting magnets.

Short term exposure to static magnetic field of the orthodontic magnets in the current study, 48 hours exposure, causes significant DNA fragmentation of the cultured human lymphocyte cells. Our finding was not in accordance with that of Bondemark et al. [16] in which they stated that "Short-term exposure to a static magnetic field did not cause any cytotoxic effect on the cells".

In current study it was concluded that, the static magnetic field per se could not dramatically induced DNA fragmentation of the living human lymphocyte cells, except in the presence of trace amounts of ferrous ions. In accordance we can't exclude the possibility of the corrosion products especially iron, from the orthodontic magnets during clinical use, to be the contributing factor for the observed cytotoxic in vitro and biological in vivo effects of the static magnetic field. The conclusion of Donohue et al. [24] added more support to the combined effect of the magnets, they stated that their results "supports the hypothesis that these are cytotoxic effects of possibly corrosion products and of magnetism" and continued "With the evidence of a biological effect, the use of implanted magnets must at present be limited until the safety can be assured".

The findings of Linder-Aronson et al. [25] in which they concluded that "It cannot be excluded that the magnetic field or corrosion products from the magnetic material influenced vital processes in the epithelium and the bone close to the magnets" gives more strong evidence to our findings. On the other hand Miyakoshi [26] stated that "It has also been reported that treatment with trace amounts of ferrous ions in the cell culture medium and exposure to a static magnetic field increases DNA damage, which is detected using the comet assay".

One of the most important finding of the current study is that; static magnetic field of orthodontic magnets per se had no significant effects on the cultured human lymphocyte cells. On the other hand, adding traces of iron to the cell culture medium enhancing the effects of static magnetic field on the cultured cells. This result give support to the conclusion in previous clinical study by the authors in which they stated that the DNA fragmentation of the oral mucosa cells on the magnets' side was significantly higher than that reported on the non-magnets' side [27].

The adverse biological effects of the static magnetic field of orthodontic magnets, recorded in the current study, in the form of DNA fragmentation of human lymphocyte cells, ring the bill so that orthodontic magnets should be used with great care in orthodontic practice among other dental and medical specialties till more complete understanding of this vital serious issue has been established.

Conclusion

The data of the current study was interpreted and discussed in view of the available literature and the following conclusions and recommendations had been extracted:

1. Exposure to static magnetic field of the commercial orthodontic samarium-cobalt (SmCo5) magnets, for only 48 hours induces significant DNA fragmentation of human lymphocyte cells.
2. The adverse biological effect of exposing vital human lymphocyte cells to the static magnetic field of orthodontic magnets fixed in attractive mode is significantly higher compared to that of magnets fixed in repelling mode.
3. Iron is a significant factor to enhance the destructive effects of the static magnetic field of orthodontic magnets on vital cells.

Recommendation

1. Under such circumstances it is highly recommended to be cautious with the wide spread use of magnets in orthodontic practice, in particular, and in dentistry and other medical specialties in general, till this critical and crucial issue will be completely investigated, other wise the whole subject will be medicolegally completely prohibited.
2. The results of the current study encourage other researchers to develop long-term stable protective magnets coats strong enough to withstand the unpredictable oral environmental changes during clinical uses, in such way that it will prevent metal ions release especially iron ion from orthodontic magnets.

References

[1] Gianelly A, Vaitas A, Thomas W. The use of magnets to move molars distally. *Am. J. Orthod. Dentofac. Orthop.* 1989; 96: 161 -7.

[2] Bondemark L, Kurol J. Distalization of maxillary first and second molars simultaneously with repelling magnets. *Eur. J. Orthod.* 1992; 14: 264-72.

[3] Sandler PJ. An attractive solution to unerupted teeth. *Am. J. Orthod. Dentofac. Orthop.* 1991; 100: 489-93.

[4] Vardimon A, Graber TM, Drescher D, Bourauel C. Rare earth magnets and impaction. Am J Orthod Dentofac Orthop 1991; 100:494-512. Vardimon A, Graber TM, Drescher D, Bourauel C. Rare earth magnets and impaction. *Am. J. Orthod. Dentofac. Orthop.* 1991; 100:494-512.

[5] Darendeliler MA, Freidle JM. Treatment of an impacted canine with magnets. *J. Clinic Orthod.* 1994; 28: 639-42.

[6] Springate SD, Sandler PJ. Micro-magnetic retainer: an attractive solution to fixed retention. *Br. J. Orthod.* 1991; 18: 139-41.

[7] Drandelier MA, Yuksel S, Meral O. Open-bite correction with magnetic activator device. *J. Clin. Orthod.* 1995; 9: 569-76.

[8] Kiliaridis S, Egermark I, Thilander B. Anterior open bite treatment with magnets. *Eur. J. Orthod.* 1990; 12:447-57.

[9] Vardimon AD, Graber TM, Voss LR, Verrusio E. Magnetic versus mechanical expansion with different force thresholds and points of application. *Am. J. Orthod. Dentofac. Orthop.* 1987; 92: 455-66.

[10] Vardimon AD, Graber TM, Voss LR, Muller TP. Functional orthopedic appliance (FOMA) III-Modus operandi. *Am. J. Orthod. Dentofac. Orthop.* 1990; 97; 135-48.

[11] Karla V, Burstone C, Nanda R. Effects of a fixed magnetic appliance on the dentofacial complex. *Am. J. Orthod. Dentofac. Orthop.* 1989; 95:467-78.

[12] Tsutsui H, Kinouchi Y, Sasaki H, Shiota M, Ushita T. Studies on the Sm-Co magnet as a dental material. *J. Dent. Res.* 1979; 58: 1597-606.

[13] Costello J, Pratten J, Evans R, Noar J. The corrosion of rare earth orthodontic magnets. *J. Orthod.* 2000; 27: 111-12.

[14] Mikloš M, Gajski G, Garaj – Vrhovac V. Usage of the standard and modified comet assay in assessment of DNA damage in human lymphocytes after exposure to ionizing radiation. *Radiol. Oncol. 2009*; 43(2): 97-107.

[15] Papadopulos M, Hoerler I, Gerber B, Rahn B, Rakosi T. Biologic effects of static magnetic fields on osteoblast cells in culture. *Eur. J. Orthod.* 1990; 12: 507-21.

[16] McDonald F. Effect of static magnetic fields on osteoblasts and fibroblasts in vitro. *Bioelectromagnetics* 1993; 14: 187-96.

[17] Papadopoulos MA. Biological aspects of the use of permanent magnets and static magnetic fields in Orthodontics. *Hellenic Orthodontic Review* 1998; 1:145-57.

[18] Yamamoto Y, Ohsaki Y, Goto T, Nakasima A, Iijima T. Effects of static magnetic fields on bone formation in rat osteoblast cultures. *J. Dent. Res.* 2003; 82: 962-6.

[19] Camilleri S, McDonald F. The effect of static magnetic fields on sutural cellular proliferation. *Eur. J. Orthod.* 1990; 12: 490.

[20] Camilleri S, McDonald F. Static magnetic field effect on the sagittal suture in Rattus Norvegicus. *Am. J. Orthod. Dentofacial Orthop.* 1993; 103: 240-6.

[21] Bondemark L , Kurol J, Wisten A. Extent and flux density of static magnetic fields generated by orthodontic samarium-cobalt magnets. *Am. J. Orthod. Dentofac. Orthop.* 1995; 107: 488-96.

[22] Miyakoshi J. The review of cellular effects of a static magnetic field. *Science and Technology of Advanced Materials.* 2006; 7: 305–307.

[23] Raylman RR, Clavo AC, Wahl RL. Exposure to strong static magnetic field slows the growth of human cancer cells in vitro. *Bioelectromagnetics.* 1996; 17(5):358-63.

[24] Donohue VE, McDonald F, Evans R. In vitro cytotoxicity testing of neodymium-iron-boron magnets. *J. Appl. Biomater.* 1995; 6:69–74.

[25] Linder-Aronson S, Lindskog S. A morphometric study of bone surfaces and skin reactions after stimulation with static magnetic fields in rats. *Am. J. Orthod. Dentofacial Orthop.* 1991;99:44–8.

[26] Miyakoshi J. Effects of static magnetic fields at the cellular level. *Prog. Biophys. Mol. Biol.* 2005; 87(2-3):213-23.

[27] Abdel-Kader HM, Aref MI, Hussein FA. Coating Failure of Commercial Orthodontic Magnets and DNA Fragmentation in Oral Mucosa Cells. *AOJ* 2008: 24; 32-40.

In: A Window on Surgery and Orthodontics
Editor: Giuseppe Alessandro Scardina

ISBN: 978-1-62808-948-6

Chapter XIV

Temporo-Mandibular Joint Reconstruction with Alloplastic Prostheses in the TMJ Ankylosis: Our Experience

Mercurio Alessandra[1], Andrea Braconi[1*], Francesco Noto[1] and Luigi Solazzo

[1]Division of Maxillofacial Surgery, ARNAS Civico,
Di Cristina e Benfratelli, Palermo, Italy

Abstract

Aim. The treatment of temporomandibular joint (TMJ) ankylosis aims to eliminate the neoformed tissue and to re-establish the mandibular functionality. The purpose of this article is to evaluate the best surgical treatment considering the complications, the functional and aesthetic aspect, through a retrospective study carried out on nine patients treated by resection of ankylosed bone followed by reconstruction with a total joint prosthesis.

Methods. From June 2003 to June 2009, nine patients presenting with temporomandibular ankylosis underwent a surgical reconstruction of the TMJ by employing a "Quinn prosthesis", at the Department of Maxillary-Facial Surgery of the "Civico" Hospital in Palermo. Among them, 7 were male (25 to 50 years old with a mean age of 42,3) and 2 were female (37 and 54 years old and the mean age was 45,5).

Results. In the considered sample of patients the mean preoperative maximum interincisal distance was 6,6 mm, this was increased to a mean of 32 mm postoperatively. Only one patient developed an infection postoperatively.

* Address correspondence and reprint requests to: Andrea Braconi, MD, Via Fr. Scaduto n.12, 90144 Palermo, Italy, Mob: +39 338 7000865. e-mail: a_braconi@hotmail.com.

Conclusions. The authors concluded that reconstruction with a total alloplastic joint prosthesis has proven to lead to successful outcomes in the management of severe anatomic joint disease in adult patients.

Keywords: Temporomandibular joint prosthesis, TMJ reconstruction, TMJ replacement, ankylosis, Quinn prosthesis

Introduction

Temporal mandibular joint ankylosis stands for irreversible, total or partial immobility of joint capsules due to anatomic alterations of the very joint components.

Ankylosis is chiefly subdivided into intra and extra-articular, mono and bilateral ankylosis [1-2]. Intra-articular ankylosis is characterized by a more or less complete upsetting of the TMJ leading to the disappearance of the articular chamber, moreover, extra-articular ankylosis differs from the other types of ankylosis as it involves the adjacent anatomic structures.

Ankylosis may be defined as complete or incomplete depending on the variable extent of the ankylotic block. The latter may progressively involve, besides the condyle, the glenoid cavity, the tympanic bone, the coronoid process, the sigmoid incisure and the zygomatic bone.

The etiopathogenesis recognizes three possible causes: traumatic, infectious and some systemic disease [3]. Traumatic events represent the most reported cause of ankylosis [4]. The hypothesis has been proposed that in cases caused by trauma, intra-articular haematoma, scarring and excessive bone formation give rises to hypomobility.

A variety of techniques for treatment of ankylosis have been described in the literature. However, no single method has produced uniformly successful results. In this paper, we describe an approach to the treatment of TMJ ankylosis that includes: 1) resection of the ankylosed bone, 2) coronoidectomy, 3) reconstruction TMJ with a total alloplastic joint prostheses.

Material and Methods

Between 2003 and 2011, nine patients, presenting with temporomandibular ankylosis, were treated by resection of ankylosed bone, followed by reconstruction with a total joint prosthesis (total twelve Quinn prosthesis) at the Department of Maxillary-Facial Surgery of the "Civico" Hospital in Palermo. Data concerning age, sex, aetiology, joint affected were collected. The preoperative assessment included a detailed patient history and physical examination. The degree of limitation of mouth opening was assessed by measuring maximum interincisal opening with a caliper.

Investigations for all patients included ortopantomography and CT scans of the maxillo-facial bones.

Surgical Technique

Patients were operated upon general anesthesia using nasotracheal intubation. The surgical approach to the joint was in all cases via pre-auricolar and submandibular approach. The surgical protocol was as follows: 1) resection of ankylosed bone; 2) ipsilateral coronoidectomy; 3) reconstruction with a total joint prosthesis.

The TMJ was approached using two incisions: a) preauricolar incision with a 1. 5 to 2 cm extension into the temporal hair-line for exposure of the temporalis fascia; b) sub-mandibular incision. The dissection proceeded to the zygomatic arch and extended anteriorly and posteriorly to expose the ankylosed TMJ. After exposure and identification of the site of ankylosis, aggressive excision of bony mass was carried out. The critical surgical elements included adeguate resection of the ankylosed parts of the joint and creation of a gap of 2 - 3 cm between the remaining portion of the mandibular ramus and the glenoid fossa. The coronoid process was resected. Once the fossa components of both sides were placed and fixated, the patient was placed in the post-operatory intermaxillary relationship, which was secured with wire fixation. A Quinn prosthesis was used as a spacer to prevent reankylosis. Condylar prosthesis was designed to replace the articular surface of the mandibular condyle.

The mandibular prosthesis is made of Cobalt Chromium alloy. The fossa prosthesis is designed to replace the articulating surface of the temporomandibular joint comprised of the glenoid fossa and the articular eminence of the temporal bone. The fossa made of Arcom ultra high molecular weight polyethylene. The system screws are made of 6AL/4L titanium.

Results

Our sample included 7 males (25 to 50 years old with a mean age of 42,3) and 2 females (37 and 54 years old and the mean age was 45,5). Six patients had unilateral and three had bilateral ankylosis (an illustrative case of bilateral ankylosis treatment can be seen in Figure 1). The mean preoperative maximum interincisal distance was 6,6 (range 5,3 – 11 mm), wich was increased to a mean of 32 mm postoperatively. The causes of ankylosis were trauma in all 9 cases. Common to all patients was the inability to open the mouth, malocclusion with poor oral hygiene. Follow-up of the 9 patients has been between 2 and 8 years.

In all patients, the maximum intercisal distance increased significantly following surgery and remained stable at the 2 year control (mean 32, min 27mm, max 37 mm).

One patient developed an infection five days post-operatively. Two patients developed a salivary fistula with spontaneous resolution. No recurrence was observed in our series.

Discussion

Management of temporomandibular joint ankylosis requires a combination of surgery and early physioterapy to restore mandibular function and prevent recurrence [5].

Following the first condylectomy [6], advances in the technique have developed three fundamental points: recurrences prevention, reconstructive phase and functional rehabilitation. Precocious physiotherapy and the choice of interposition material represent the most important requirements for recurrence prevention. The meticulous and radical elimination of the ankylosis was recommended by Raveh et al. (1989) [7] and Kaban (1990) [8]: an incomplete removal of the ankylosed bone would lead to re-ankylosis especially in the medial aspect of the joint. Sophisticated reconstruction is needed for such total resection of the joint to provide rehabilitation of mandibular movement, restore mandibular ramus height, improve the occlusal plane.

Separation of the cut bone surfaces may be accomplished by utilizing muscle, pedicled temporalis and masseter muscle, fascia lata, full thickness skin, autogenous cartilage, lyophilized dura, methyl methacrylate, silicone, teflon, autologus costocondral grafts, and prefabricated joint prostheses [9-21]. However, there are possible disadvantages, such as morbidity at the donor site and unpredictable resorption when autogenous material is used, and a risk of foreign body reaction when alloplastic material is used. The following problems are encountered with present grafts: muscle shrinkage and fibroses, fascia lacking bulk, cartilage tending to fibrose and calcify, and alloplastic implants under functional loads disintegrating and causing foreign body giant cell reactions.

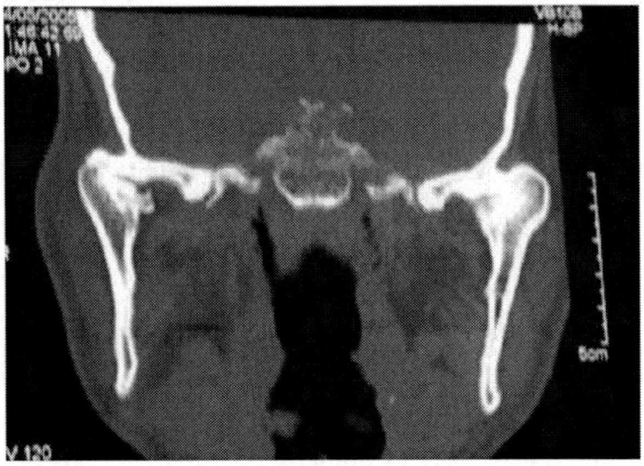

Figure 1a). Coronal view of a CT scan showing a bilateral TMJ ankylosis.

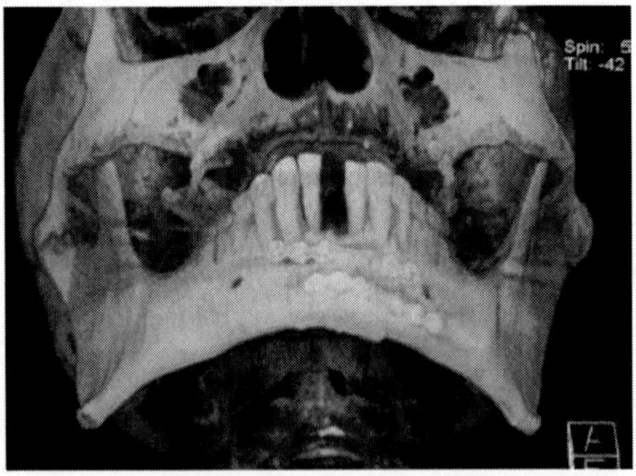

Figure 1b). Volume Rendering CT showing the bilateral TMJ ankylosis and the outcome of a previous surgical treatment for a maxilla-mandibular trauma.

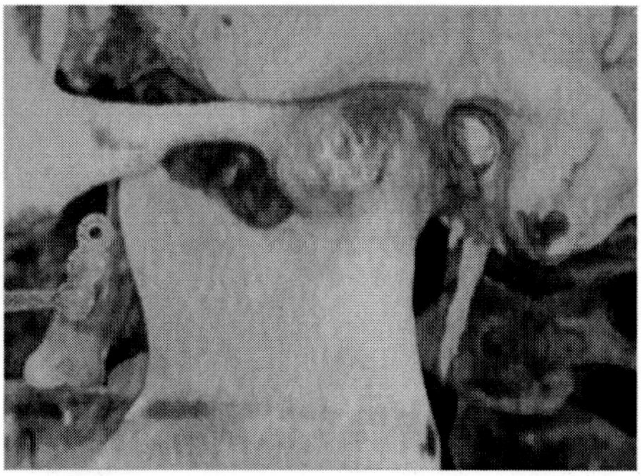

Figure 1c). Volume Rendering CT of the left TMJ ankylosis.

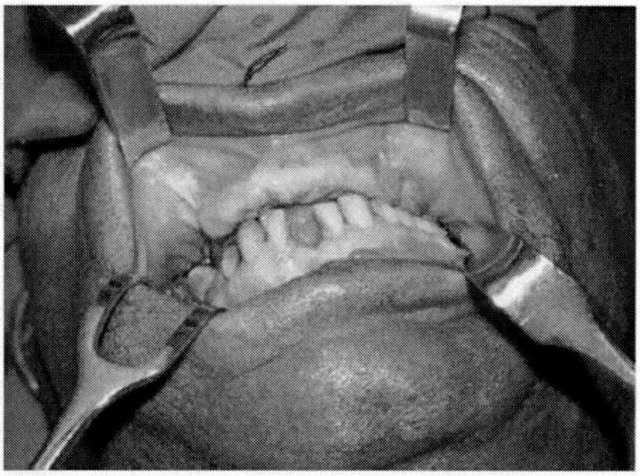

Figure 1d). Intraoperative view of maximum oral opening.

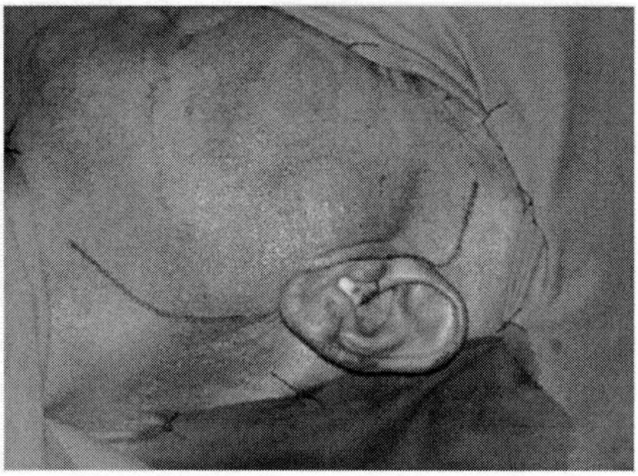

Figure 1e). Incision lines marked preoperatively.

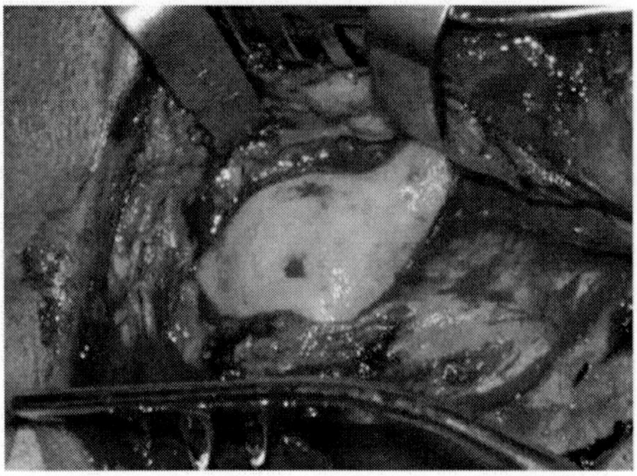

Figure 1f). Exposition of the left ankylotic block.

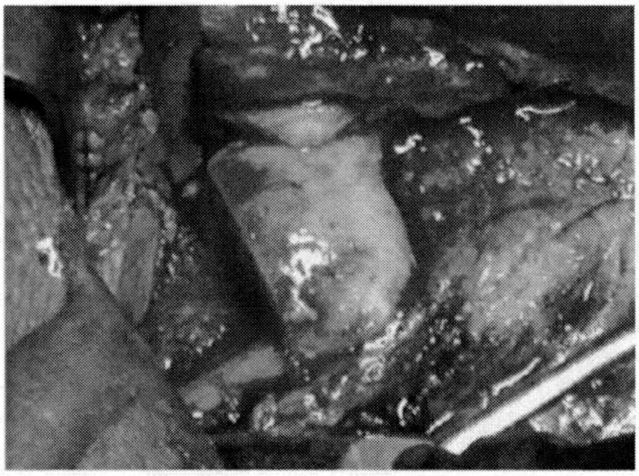

Figure 1g). Surgical field after the removal of the left ankylotic block.

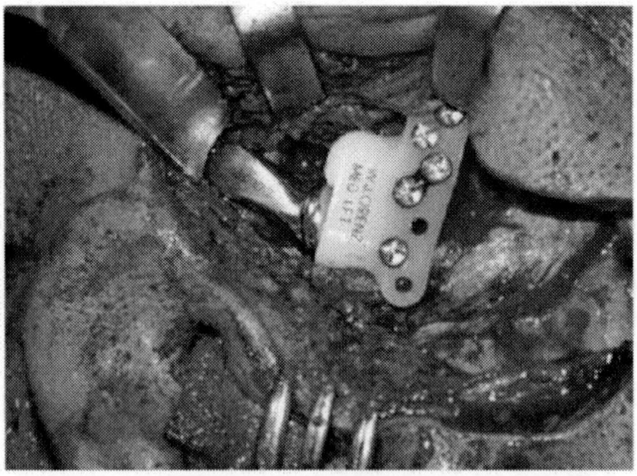

Figure 1h). Surgical field after the placement of the Quinn prosthesis. View through preauricolar exposition.

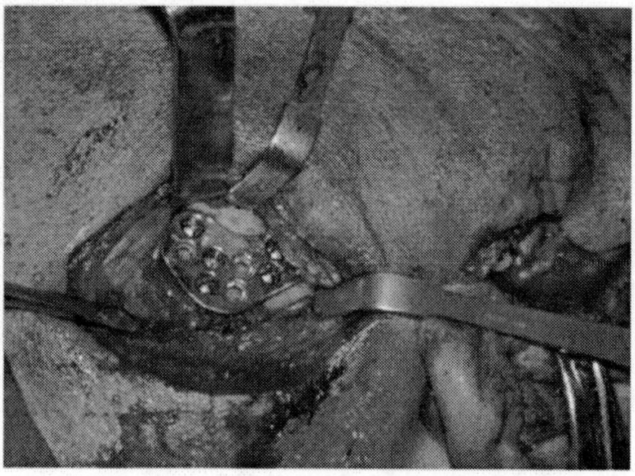

Figure 1i). Surgical field after the placement of the Quinn prosthesis. View through submandibular exposition.

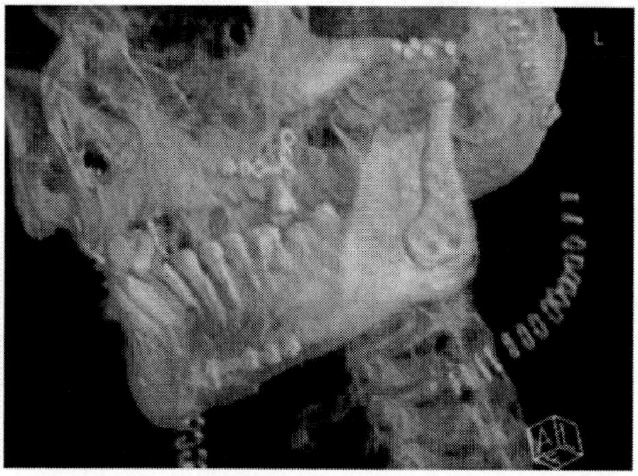

Figure 1j). Postoperative Volume rendering CT of the left TMJ.

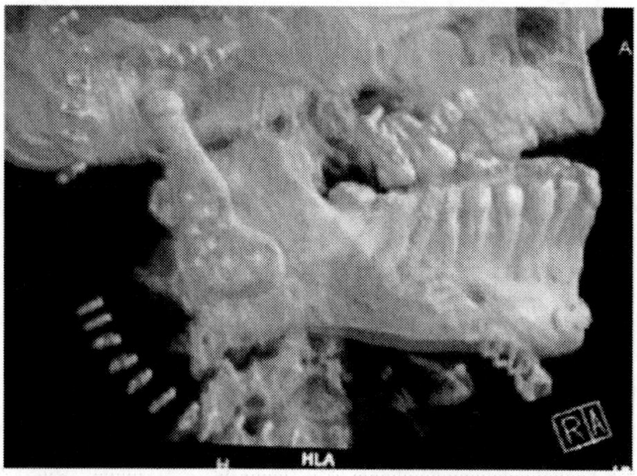

Figure 1k). Postoperative Volume rendering CT of the right TMJ.

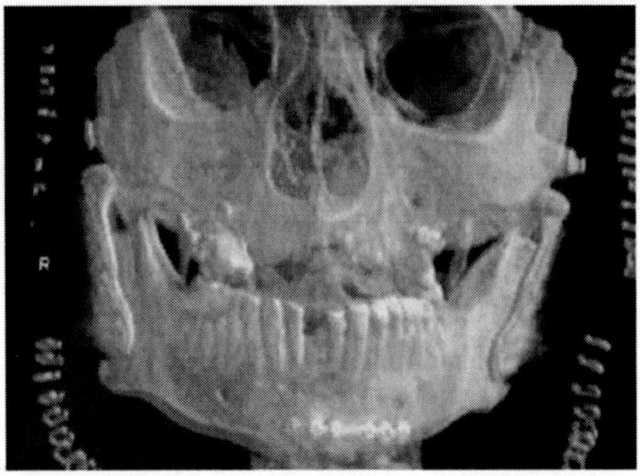

Figure 1l). Postoperative Volume rendering CT both the TMJ.

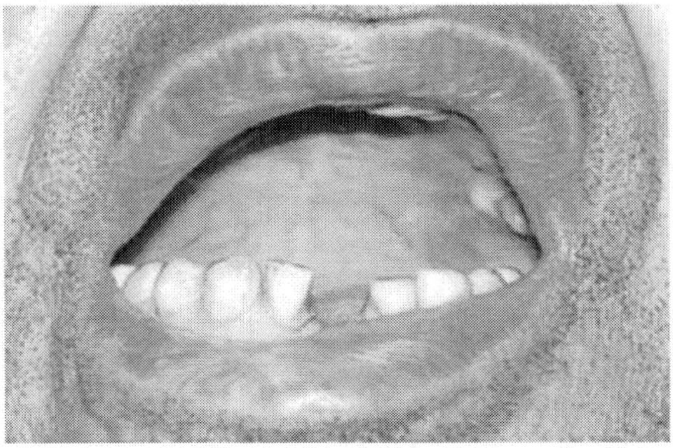

Figure 1m). Postoperative view of maximum oral opening.

Among the alloplastic materials, the proplast/Teflon and the silastic have been widely used in the 80 in order to treat TMJ disorders such as synovial condromatosis, osteoarthiritis as well as ankylosis.

Further studies on the long term results of these materials, have highlighted the failure of alloplastic implantations. Following surgical treatment of the recurrence , an istopathological analysis was performed which elucidated tha presence of histiocyte accumulation in immediate contact with silicate particles, of phagocytes in the intracellular material and lymphocyte T in the vicinity of silicate particle. Over time, these cellular reactions results into the neoformation of intraarticular tissue with clinical evidence of recurrence and, in any way, into the persistent limitation of mandibular functionally.

In this study, however, no patient was treated with interpositional graft.

Today, alloplastic TMJ replacement can be categorized into prosthesis providing replacement of the fossa only, prosthesis and reconstruction plates for replacement of the condyle, and prosthesis for the combined replacement of the fossa and the condyle[22]. Alloplastic joints are said to allow a closer reproduction of the normal anatomy of the joint, with restoration of vertical dimension, avoidance of donor site morbidity, reduction in operation time and a lower risk of recurrent ankylosis.

Currently accepted indications for joint reconstruction are as follows [23]: massive ankylosis or reankylosis, failed autogenous graft in multiply operated patient, severe inflammatory joint disease affecting TMJ, status post-neoplasia resection.

Contraindications to the use: skeletal immaturity, systemic disease (diabetes, myelodysplasia) active infection, allergy to the materials.

Advantages to the use: immediate functional ability without prolonged intermaxillary fixation, lack of donor site morbidity, no need intermaxillary fixation and reduced intraoperative surgical time. Disadvantages: cost of prosthesis, potential wear debris and associated pathologic responses, unpredictable need for revision surgery. The long follow up of these patients proved this mode of therapy to be satisfactory.

Conclusion

The results of our study, in according to literature, showed that the TMJ prosthesis provided significantly better outcomes relative to jaw opening, pain relief, jaw function.

The authors concluded that reconstruction with a total alloplastic joint prosthesis has proven to lead to successful outcomes in the management of severe anatomic joint disease in adult patients.

References

[1] Rowe NL. Ankylosis of the temporomandibular joint. *J. R. Coll Surg. Edinb.* 1982; 27(2):67-79.

[2] Kaban LB, Perrott DH, Fisher K. A protocol for management of temporomandibular joint ankylosis. *J. Oral Maxillofac. Surg.* 1990;48:1145-51.

[3] Topazian RG. Etiology of ankylosis of the temporomandibular joint. Analysis of 44 cases. *J. Oral. Surg. Anesth Hosp. Dent. Serv.* 1964;22:227-33.

[4] Guven O. Fractures of the maxillofacial region in children. *J. Craniomaxillofac. Surg.* 1992;20(6):244-7.

[5] Cherry CQ, Frew A Jr. High condylectomy for treatment of arthritis of the temporomandibular joint. *J. Oral. Surg.* 1977; 35(4):285-8.

[6] Young AH. A follow-up of 12 cases of ankylosis of the temporal mandibular joint treated by condilectomy. *Brit. J. Plast. Surg.* 1963;16:75.

[7] Raveh J, Vuillemin T, Ladrach K, Sutter J. Temporomandibular joint ankylosis: surgical treatment and long-term results. *J. Oral Maxillofac. Surg.* 1989; 47(9):900-6.

[8] Kaban LB, Pogrel MA. The role of a temporalis fascia and muscle flap in temporomandibular joint surgery. *J. Oral Maxillofac. Surg* 1990;48:14-9.

[9] Gallagher DM, Wolford LM. Comparison of Silastic and Proplast implants in the temporomandibular joint after condylectomy for osteoarthritis. *J. Oral Maxillofac. Surg.* 1982;40:627.

[10] Meyer RA. The autogenous dermal graft in temporomandibular joint disc surgery. *J. Oral Maxillofac. Surg.* 1988;46:948-54.

[11] Matukas VJ, Lachner J. The use of autologous auricular cartilage for temporomandibular joint disc replacement: a preliminary report. *J. Oral Maxillofac. Surg.* 1990; 48:348-53.

[12] MacIntosh RB. The use of autogenous tissues for temporomandibular joint reconstruction. *J. Oral Maxillofac. Surg.* 2000;58:63-69.

[13] Chossegros C, Guyot L, Cheynet F, Blanc JL, Gola R, Bourczak Z, Conrath J. Comparison of different materials for interposition arthroplasty in treatment of temporomandibular joint ankylosis surgery: long-term follow-up in 25 cases. *Br. J. Oral Maxillofac. Surg.* 1997;35: 157-60.

[14] Pogrel M. A., Kaban LB. The role of a temporalis fascia and muscle flap in temporomandibular joint surgery. J. Oral Maxillofac. Surg. 1990;48:14-19.

[15] Lei Z. Auricular cartilage graft interposition after temporomandibular joint ankylosis surgery in children. *J. Oral Maxillofac. Surg.* 2002; Sep;60(9):985-7.

[16] Dimitroulis G. The interpositional dermis-fat graft in the management of temporomandibular joint ankylosis. *Int. J. Oral Maxillofac. Surg.* 2004 Dec;33(8): 755-60.

[17] Saeed NR, Kent JN. A retrospective study of the costochondral graft in TMJ reconstruction. *Int. J. Oral Maxillofac. Surg.* 2003 Dec;32(6):606-9.

[18] Mandibular joint arthrosis corrected by the insertion of a cast-Vittalium glenoid fossa prosthesis: a new tecnique. *Oral Surg.* 1964;17(6):712.

[19] Su-Gwan K. Treatment of temporomandibular joint ankylosis with temporalis muscle and fascia flap. *Int. J. Oral Maxillofac. Surg.* 2001; 30:189-93.

[20] Lei Z. Auricular cartilage graft interposition after temporomandibular joint ankylosis surgery in children. *J. Oral Maxillofac. Surg.* 2002; Sep;60(9):985-7.

[21] Manganello-Souza LC, Mariani PB. Temporomandibular joint ankylosis: report of 14 cases. *Int. J. Oral Maxillofac. Surg.* 2003 Feb;32(1):24-9.

[22] Mercuri LG. The use of alloplastic prostheses for temporomandibular joint recostruction. *J. Oral Maxillofac. Surg.* 2000;58:70-5.

[23] Peter D. Quinn. Color Atlas of Temporomandibular joint surgery. *Mosby* 1986.

In: A Window on Surgery and Orthodontics
Editor: Giuseppe Alessandro Scardina
ISBN: 978-1-62808-948-6

Chapter XV

Local Anesthetic Efficacy and Systemic Influence of 4% Articaine HCl vs. 2% Lidocaine HCl with 1:100,000 Epinephrine: A Randomized Controlled Prospective Study

Liran Levin[1]* and Shaul Lin[2]

[1]Department of Periodontology, School of Graduate Dentistry, Rambam Health Care Campus, Haifa, Israel and Harvard Scool of Dental Medicine, Boston, MA, US

[2]Endodontics and Dental Trauma Unit, School of School of Graduate Dentistry, Rambam Health Care Campus, Haifa, and Faculty of Medicine, Technion, Israel

Abstract

Aim: The purpose of this study was to evaluate the anesthetic efficacy of 4% articaine and 2% lidocaine, both containing 1:100,000 epinephrine, and the influence on heart rate during endodontic treatment.

Methodology: The study examined 244 patients requiring root canal treatment who were randomly assigned either articaine or lidocaine. Anesthetic efficacy was evaluated by the need for additional injections and by self-perceived information on pain reported at several time points on a Visual Analogue Scale (VAS) (total pain perception, pain during injection, and pain during treatment). Heart rate was electronically measured before treatment, during injection, and during treatment.

Results: Lidocaine was administered to 128 patients and articaine to 116. No statistical difference was found in the requirement for additional injections. The articaine

* Correspondence and reprints to: Correspondence and reprint requests to: Dr. Liran Levin, Department of Periodontology, School of Graduate Dentistry, Rambam Health Care Campus, Haifa, Israel, Fax: +972-4-85431717; E-mail: liranl@technion.ac.il.

group reported less pain on VAS at all time points (p<0. 005). A statistically significant difference was observed in heart rate after lidocaine (84. 63 beats/min) compared to articaine (81. 63 beats/min) (p=0. 048).

Conclusion: Articaine resulted in less self-reported pain during endodontic treatment.

Keywords: Pain, heart rate, anasthesia, dental surgery, anxiety

Introduction

Since 2000, articaine hydrochloride, formulated as a 4% solution containing 1:100,000 epinephrine, has been widely available in the United States [1]. Articaine possesses a unique structure, containing both an amide linkage in its intermediate chain and an ester side chain on a thiophene ring [2]. The rapid conversion of this ester moiety to a carboxylic acid moiety in the bloodstream accounts for the relatively short half-life of the drug [3] and possibly an enhanced systemic safety profile compared with that of other dental local anesthetic solutions [4]. Adequate local anesthesia is a critical component of successful patient management in endodontic therapy. Articaine appears to provide a longer lasting pulpal anesthesia than lidocaine [5, 6].

Mechanisms contributing to the difficulty of obtaining pulpal anesthesia in teeth with irreversible pulpitis have been described [7, 8]. Supplemental injections (with different techniques and/or types of anesthesia) are frequently required in patients with irreversible pulpitis, primarily because pulpal anesthesia resulting from an initial injection is often inadequate to complete the endodontic procedures [7-10]. The effect of a mandibular intra-osseous injection of 2% lidocaine with 1:100,000 epinephrine has been assessed on heart rate and blood pressure of 20 volunteer patients [11]. Changes in blood pressure from pre-operative levels were minimal and did not vary significantly at any time of measurement. The only statistically significant change in heart rate occurred immediately after the intra-osseous injection. In another report, 80% of the subjects had a mean increase in heart rate of 23-24 beats per minute with the intra-osseous injection of mepivacaine and lidocaine. There were no significant differences between results with the two solutions [12]. When cardiovascular safety profiles of articaine and lidocaine solution were compared in cardiovascular patients, no statistically significant differences were found between the two groups in heart rate, systolic or diastolic blood pressure, and/or oxygen saturation [13].

The purpose of this prospective, randomized, controlled study was to evaluate the anesthetic efficacy of 4% articaine and 2% lidocaine, both containing 1:100,000 epinephrine, as well as the effect on heart rate during endodontic treatment.

Materials and Methods

The study group consisted of 244 patients (93 men - 38. 1%; 151 women - 61. 9%) referred for endodontic treatment between January 2007 and March 2008 and treated by one endodontic specialist. Patients ranged in age from 20 to 80 years (average 47. 5±13. 8 years).

All patients presented with a single tooth requiring root canal treatment. Medical history, age, gender, and the tooth involved were recorded. Excluded were patients with systemic cardiovascular disease and/or diabetes. The Ethics Committee of Tel Aviv University approved the study. Patients signed a consent statement. Before treatment, patients were randomly divided into one of two local anesthetic groups, either 4% articaine HCl or 2% lidocaine HCl, both with 1:100,000 epinephrine. A single operator (SL) administered all local anesthetic injections (1. 8 ml) in the mucobuccal fold adjacent to the treated tooth using a standard dental aspirating syringe fitted with a 30-gauge needle. Injections were administered at a rate of 0. 9 ml per 15 s. Randomization was determined using a computer-generated sequence of random numbers. Patients were asked to rate their pain level and discomfort using a standard visual analogue scale (VAS) [14] with endpoints tagged "no pain" (0 cm) to "unbearable pain" (10 cm). Pain was assessed overall, during initial anesthetic injection, and during treatment. An electrical heart beat (Pulse Oximeter, Smiths Medical International Limited, Watford, UK) measuring device recorded the heart rate before initial treatment, during initial anesthetic injection, and during treatment. Student's t-test and Pearson's correlation and SPSS 12. 0 (SPSS, Inc., Chicago, IL, USA) were used for descriptive analysis. Statistical significance was set at the probability level of $p<0.05$.

Results

Lidocaine was administered to 128 (52. 5%) and articaine to 116 (47. 5%) patients. Tooth distribution included incisors (12. 7%), premolars (28. 7%) and molars (58. 6%), in both the mandibular (46. 3%) and maxillary (53. 7%).

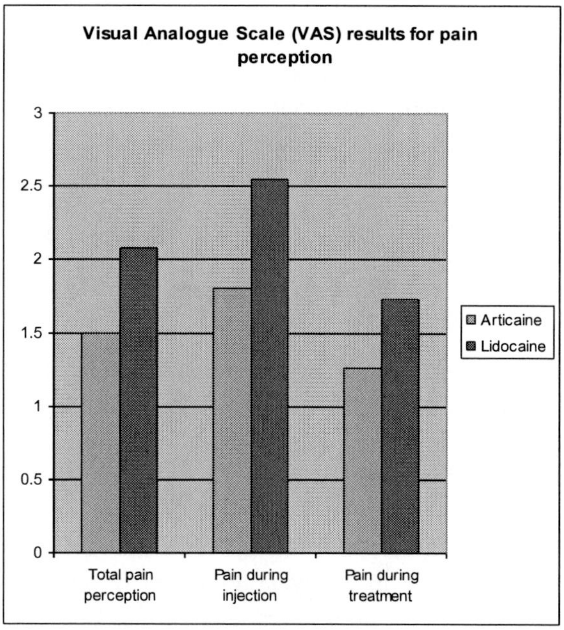

$p<0.005$.

Figure 1. Visual Analogue Scale (VAS) results for pain perception.

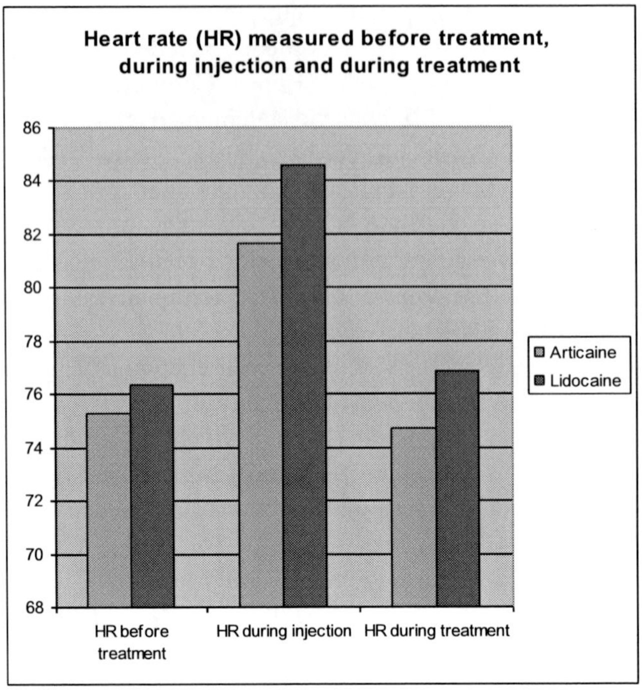

*p=0. 048.

Figure 2. Heart rate measured before treatment, during injection, and during treatment.

There was no statistical difference in the requirement for additional injections between groups. Figure 1 presents the mean VAS pain grading of patients at the different times of evaluation. Patients in the articaine group graded their pain to be lower on VAS scale at all time points, i. e., overall, during initial anesthetic injection, and during treatment (p<0. 005). Heart rate measured before treatment, during injection, and during treatment is presented in Figure 2. A statistically significant difference in heart rate was observed after lidocaine injection (84. 63 beats/min) compared to articaine injection (81. 63 beats/min) (p=0. 048). No statistically significant difference in heart rate was observed before and during treatment.

Discussion

During dental treatment, pain control is important, since an individual's pain experience is often a determinant as to whether patients will seek health care when needed [15, 16]. Local anesthetics are essential for successful endodontic treatment, and their pharmacologic characteristics have special implications for treating painful, chronically-inflamed, or necrotic teeth [17].

Recently, Kanaa et al. [18] found that for buccal infiltration of the mandibular first molar, 4% articaine with 1:100,000 epinephrine, was significantly better than 2% lidocaine with 1:100,000 epinephrine. However, the anesthetic success rate was only 64% for the articaine solution, which does not provide predictable pulpal anesthesia for all patients requiring profound anesthesia. In another study, the success rate for maxillary buccal infiltration to produce pulpal anesthesia was 100% in the first premolar and first molar with articaine compared to lidocaine (80% in the first premolar and 30% in the first molar) [19]. There was a highly significant difference between the solutions. According to the above studies, as well as the present one, the efficacy of 4% articaine is superior to 2% lidocaine for local anesthesia.

The relationship between inferior alveolar nerve block injections with articaine and an increased incidence of prolonged dysaesthesia has been shown in several case reports [20, 21]. The use of articaine in mandibular block analgesia causes more frequent lingual nerve injury than inferior alveolar nerve injury. All grades of neurosensory and gustatory functional loss have been found, as well as a range of persisting neurogenic malfunctions. Subjective complaints and neurosensory function tests indicate that lingual nerve lesions are more incapacitating than inferior alveolar nerve lesions [22]. This adverse effect, though uncommon, should be further assessed in large scale studies. In the current study, this event was not reported. The quantification of pain through use of a standard VAS pain scale does not fully predict the clinical efficacy of different anesthetics .A patient with a lower VAS score after injection might require an additional rescue injection. In contrast, a patient with a higher VAS score after injection might not require a further rescue injection.

The patient's clinical response may be modified by non-odontogenic factors, which include gender, ethnicity, genetics, emotional, and physiological factors (7). The clinician's approach to the patient may also be a significant variable.

Conclusion

Local infiltration of 4% articaine with 1:100,000 epinephrine resulted in less self-reported pain than 2% lidocaine during endodontic treatment.

References

[1] U. S. Food and Drug Administration, Center for Drug Evaluation and Research (2008) FDA drug approvals list. Available at: "www. fda. gov/cder/da/da.htm". Accessed August 13, 2008.

[2] Malamed SF, Gagnon S, Leblanc D (2000) Efficacy of articaine: a new amide local anesthetic. *Journal of the American Dental Association* 131, 635-42.

[3] Oertel R, Rahn R, Kirch W (1997) Clinical pharmacokinetics of articaine. *Clinical Pharmacokinetics* 33, 417-25.

[4] Vree TB, Gielen MJ (2005) Clinical pharmacology and the use of articaine for local and regional anaesthesia. *Best Practical Research in Clinical Anaesthesiology* 19, 293-308.

[5] Costa CG, Tortamano IP, Rocha RG, Francischone CE, Toramano N (2005) Onset and duration periods of articaine and lidocaine on maxillary infiltration. *Quintessence International* 36, 197-201.

[6] Oliveira PC, Volpato MC, Ramacciato JC, Ranali J (2004) Articaine and lidocaine efficiency in filtration anesthesia: a pilot study. *British Dental Journal* 197, 45-6.

[7] Hargreaves KM (2001) Neurochemical factors in injury and inflammation in orofacial tissues. In: Lavigne G, Lund J, Sessle B, Dubner R, eds. *Orofacial Pain: Basic Sciences to Clinical Management*. Chicago: Quintessence Publications.

[8] Walton R, Torabinejad M. Managing local anesthesia problems in the endodontic patient. *Journal of the American Dental Association* 123, 97-102.

[9] Cohen HP, Cha BY, Spangberg LS (1993) Endodontic anesthesia in mandibular molars: a clinical study. *Journal of Endodontics* 19, 370-3.

[10] Nusstein J, Reader A, Nist R, Beck M, Weaver J (1997) Anesthetic efficacy of the supplemental intraosseous injection of 3% mepivacaine in irreversible pulpitis. *Oral Surgery, Oral Medicine, Oral Pathology, Oral Radiology and Endodontology* 84, 676-82.

[11] Chamberlain TM, Davis RD, Murchison DF, Hansen SR, Richardson BW (2000) Systemic effects of an intraosseous injection of 2% lidocaine with 1:100,000 epinephrine. *General Dentistry* 48, 299-302.

[12] Guglielmo A, Reader A, Nist R, Beck M, Weaver J (1999) Anesthetic efficacy and heart rate effects of the supplemental intraosseous injection of 2% mepivacaine with 1:20,000 levonordefrin. *Oral Surgery, Oral Medicine, Oral Pathology, Oral Radiology and Endodontology* 87, 284-93.

[13] Elad S, Admon D, Kedmi M, *et al.* (2008) The cardiovascular effect of local anesthesia with articaine plus 1:200,000 adrenalin versus lidocaine plus 1:100,000 adrenalin in medically compromised cardiac patients: a prospective, randomized, double blinded study. *Oral Surgery, Oral Medicine, Oral Pathology, Oral Radiology and Endodontology* 105, 725-30.

[14] Huskinsson EC (1974) Measurement of pain. *Lancet* 9, 1127-31.

[15] Levin L, Amit A, Ashkenazi M (2006) Post-operative pain and use of analgesic agents following various dental procedures. *American Journal of Dentistry* 19, 245-7 .

[16] Berggren U, Pierce CJ, Eli I (2000) Characteristics of adult dentally fearful individuals. A cross-cultural study. *European Journal of Oral Science* 108, 268-74 .

[17] Jeske AH (2003) Local anesthetics: special considerations in endodontics. *Texas Dental Journal* 120, 231-7 .

[18] Kanaa MD, Whitworth JM, Corbett IP, Meechan JG (2006) Articaine and lidocaine mandibular buccal infiltration anesthesia: a prospective randomized double-blind crossover study. *Journal of Endodontics* 32, 296-8.

[19] Srinivasan N, Kavitha M, Loganathan CS, Padmini G (2009) Comparison of anesthetic efficacy of 4% articaine and 2% lidocaine for maxillary buccal infiltration in patients with irreversible pulpitis. *Oral Surgery, Oral Medicine, Oral Pathology, Oral Radiology and Endodontology* 107, 133-6.

[20] Haas DA, Lennon D (1995) A 21 year retrospective study of reports of paraesthesia following local anaesthetic administration. *Journal of the Canadian Dental Association* 61, 319-30.

[21] van Eden SP, Patel MF (2002) Prolonged paraesthesia following inferior alveolar nerve block using Articaine. *British Journal of Oral and Maxillofacial Surgery* 40, 519-20.

[22] Hillerup S, Jensen R (2006) Nerve injury caused by mandibular block analgesia. *International Journal of Oral and Maxillofacial Surgery* 35, 876-7.

Editor Contact Information

Giuseppe Alessandro Scardina, Ph.D.
Department of Surgical and Oncological Disciplines
Section of Oral Science
"G. Messina" University of Palermo
Via Del Vespro, 129-90127 PalermoItaly
E-mail 1: intjclindent@gmail.com
E-mail 2: scardina@odonto.unipa.it

Index

#

A

B

C

D

E

F

G

H

I

J

L

M

N

O

P

S

T